P.S.2027
Published
7 Earlsmere Drive, Ardsley, Barnsley S71 5HH

First Published 2000
Copyright   Ruth Hamshaw 2000
ISBN 0-9526900-9-8
Sketches by Joanne Ellison

Printed by: Dearne Valley Printers Ltd
Wath-on-Dearne, Rotherham

CONTENTS

PROLOGUE

I never wanted to be a nurse!. My mother had tentatively broached the subject to me when I was in my early teens. This idea had been forcefully rejected. "Mother" I cried, "I hate sick people, you know I do, I can't stand them".

This was explained by the very limited knowledge I had of them. My only excursion into these reaches had been when my father had taken me as a small child to see an elderly aunt whom he had expectations. She was sat up in a double bed with the inevitable steam tent. The windows were closed and curtains hung in front of the doors. The room had a permanent odour of commodes, Friars Balsam, menthol and all the stuffy smells connected with the annual attack of bronchitis. I have thought since that she was hibernating like Badger in "Wind in the Willows".

As a small child, I had another ridiculous idea which originated from having seen an old nurse (who had attended to my mother) hang a variety of her own underclothes on the line, these included woollen combinations and flannel petticoats. Consequently for many years I thought that all nurses wore these horrors.

At the time, my mother let the matter slide, but later on, after many adventures into worker's world, I suddenly came to the conclusion that I was getting nowhere and perhaps my mother was right. SHE WAS!

From the first day, even though tempted many times to give it up, fate and circumstances decreed otherwise. How glad I am, that this was so.

I chose the hospital, merely because I had lived at one time very near this one, which was called by the name of one of the founders. William Garrett by name. This gentleman, having much of this worlds goods, decided to endow the building (having erected it) as a thanksgiving for his recovery from a long and tedious illness. As the hospital was extended, there were other patrons, who supported one or more beds. The rest of the expenses were paid for by voluntary contributions from the towns folk.

At the time I started as a probationer, times were hard. In America, the 'Wall Street Crash' was in full swing and in England, there was unemployment, dole, hunger and consequently a lot of people emigrated to the colonies. Nearly everyone suffered in one way or the other and my family were no exception.

As soon as I told my mother of my decision, she took steps to see that I did not change my mind. Despite financial difficulties, she overcame these and with her usual optimism and enthusiasm, unashamedly borrowed from my grandmother. With this corn in Egypt, to back us up, I wrote for an interview and in a week or two I was on my way to London for an interview. I was notified later of the success of my application. In the meantime I had to be measured for uniform dresses of lilac linen. There were caps, collars, cuffs and white belts, also studs and black stockings (woollen or cotton).

After all these clothes had been paid for, there was not enough money left over to pay my fare. We suddenly had a brain-wave, I had a bicycle which I shared with my brother, he agreed to let me sell it and with the sum of five shillings we had raised, I just had enough cash to take me across London after I reached the city.

After many years, I can see in my minds eye, the picture of a small girl of eighteen in a red coat and a black hat, with a large case and a fair amount of self conceit setting off on the long distance bus and sweetest of all, I can see the face of my mother as she waved me goodbye. Her expressive face showing many conflicting emotions, love, pride and envy, that her eldest daughter was going to do what she had always wished.

I waved to her and the coach was soon moving and I was on my way to an adventure, which even now, twenty-eight years later is not yet finished.

CHAPTER 1
"Good Morning Nurse"

"Good morning nurse! Possess yourself of a duster, follow me, and do not deviate from the path of duty." This remark has been handed down, as a classical order, delivered to a timid and quaking probationer, on her first morning on the wards. The nurse of today may not quake, but I did.

When I presented myself at the ghastly hour of 7.30 a.m. the Staff Nurse met me at the door, took one look, and told me I had too much hair showing. While I rectified this condition, she called to a nurse, an awesome being, who in my ignorance I took to be at least the Matron. Later on I found out that she was only twenty years old, lived at Plumstead, had been at the hospital eight months, had no boyfriends, and had no hope of ever such a luxury coming her way.

For half an hour we made beds, at least, Nurse Prim made the beds and I was supposed to learn as she made. I struggled with corners, centre lines, pillows, ten inches of sheet at the top, and last but not least the inoffensive patient. It sounds easy, to talk of, but I found that we were allowed 2 minutes to make an empty bed and 3 for an occupied one. At home, beds were made for comfort, and to sleep in, but on the wards, no! they had corners, they had to be tidy, and they were like boxes made for one.

At eight o'clock sister arrived and I was taken to be introduced to her. After she had taken the report from the night sister, she introduced me to the sluice rooms. Now I had always associated this word with reservoirs, and lots of water cascading through arches. I seemed to have been misinformed, I found queer shaped sinks, with taps, which were traps for the unwary. The thing to do, was to turn it on, AFTER placing a utensil over it, this ensured that the article had "inner cleanliness." However I found that all new probates inevitably turned it on first, and it was just as though a soda syphon had been squirted. "Fetch three urinals," this I did, trying to appear as though I had been used to such kind of work all my life, I hurried to the ward door with these, held like a bunch of flowers only to be called back by sister, and told to fetch a mysterious object called a bedpan cover. This was modestly draped over the three bottles as they were known to the men.

Having been told to give each man one of these, I did so, and could not understand why some of them looked a little surprised, but meekly took them, irrespective of their needs.

Opinions varied as to the character of the sister of this male ward. Some thought she was a market of strictest type, others including the patients, thought that she was an angel, but all nurses agreed, that she was a great teacher, "her price was far above the price of rubies." (with apologies to King Solomon.)

My first impression of her was of an elderly woman in appearance, but she seemed to be supercharged with energy, and gifted with second sight.

Her hair was straight and very white, her figure non-existent. All this was redeemed by a lovely complexion and a pair of bright blue eyes. Her kindness was never ending, although her patience must have been exhausted many times.

I think she had been trained under the tuition of Florence Nightingale's pupils, and tried to bring us under the same regime, but alas, we were of another generation, and had other ideas, consequently there was bound to be a certain amount of silent disapproval.

For three months, she and the Irish staff nurse, in their separate ways, struggled with my great ignorance.

My memories of that first day on duty in this ward may be a little vague, but I know, that having started the day at 7.30 I had 2½ hours off duty from ten till twelve thirty p.m. and at 8.45 p.m. we went to supper and only then, were we allowed to go to our rooms, and thence to a bath and bed. We had to share a large room, with another Pro.

I had arrived at the hospital the evening before, and was taken to my room by the assistant Matron, who also had to do home sisters duties. She introduced me to my room companion, who I found out, had arrived only 2 hours before.

Our friendship began then, and went on all through the two years that I was there. Even afterwards when circumstances decreed that we should meet, if not often.

I had gingerly sat down on my small white bed, and Katie Susan had looked at me and grinned. She was trying to fit the pleats into the back of her cap, always a difficult procedure. I went to help her, and between us we managed to make what we thought to be a perfect model, only to be disillusioned, when the door opened and a girl, who we later knew to have the name of Georgy, short for Georgina entered. "Come on you kids, I have been sent to show you the way to the dining room. At that moment a bell rang, as though we were at school and off we went. On the way, we had a lecture from Georgina. In a patronising manner we were told that she was Senior to us, by a year and a half, and that we were to open the doors for all, who were in the enviable position to have arrived a few weeks more or less, before us.

We sat down to supper and the matron sat at the head of the table. There were about five nurses of varying ages and ranks. I took stock of Georgy, she was tall and buxom, with rosy cheeks, vivid blue eyes and very protruding teeth.

Katie Susan, was small, dark hair with a natural wave in it. She had bright brown eyes, which twinkled with fun and laughter. Her complexion was the bane of her life, it was never good, and she spent lots of time and hard earned cash trying to rectify this.

After supper we were shown the PROPER way to make up our uniform. I secretly made up my mind, that when I was used to it, I should be a lot smarter than Miss G.

I think that Katie and I rather resented the manner in which we were told that we were JUNIORS, with a capital J. But to our eternal discredit, I am afraid that we were equally patronising and dictatorial, when our time came.

I do not think that we slept at all well, on that first night we spent in hospital. We were homesick and Katie (whose surname was Mc.Lean) was openly sniffling into the pillows. She was wondering what ever made her leave The Emerald Isles.

However, just as we had gone off to sleep, there was a terrific bang on the door, it opened and a voice said, "half past six" then retreated to the next room.

We flew out of bed and struggled into the mauve linen dresses, collars, cuffs, belts, and tried to adjust our caps to a suitable angle, both becoming, and professional. You already know the result of my labour's.

Katie had a little more luck, there was no comment passed on her efforts.

Punctually at seven, there was loud clanging of the breakfast bell, and there was a rush and a flurry and Georgy appeared, with her usual cry, "Come on kids, don't be late."

We arrived at the dining room where the night sister was at the head of the table. She served bacon and eggs, marked the register, and departed. Just like school. Before she left she gave me to the care of the Irish staff nurse, and told me that I was to start my first morning on the mens ward. Katie was taken to the women's ward and I did not see her till lunch time. She told me that she was off duty from two till four thirty; this included the tea hour.

When at last we were off duty that night, we had a quick bath and each of us just fell into bed. I ached all over and thought that I was as least as ill as the patients I had seen, and Katie could only remember her "poor feet." Even her complexion took second place."

She told me that she was the daughter of a busy G. P. in a village in the north of Ireland. She, like I, was one of a fairly large family, and as fast as they were able to leave the paternal nest, they did so, as father was a doctor who at that time was more likely to be paid with a bottle of home made liquor, a chicken, a pig, vegetables, fruit, honey, but almost never did they think of cash. No…that was a commodity that was seldom seen in their house. Katie unlike me had more sisters than brothers, we swapped yarns of our respective families, I told of my four brothers, and she of her sisters. It was an endless source of conversation to us.

It was not till much time had passed, that I heard the story as it had gone, of her secret passion, (unknown and therefore unreciprocated by the object of her devotion.)

Of this, I will tell you later and what came of it.

CHAPTER 2

"In Praise Of Matrons"

The William Garrett Hospital was small and very busy. Situated on the outskirts of London, very near to a great many factories, it took in all acute cases, and the patients, apart from emergencies, were sent in and attended to by the local G.P.'s. However full up we were we never seemed to refuse anyone admission. I have seen at times of necessity, beds down the middle of the wards. This made it difficult for the nurses and made the patient feel, as one man said, "like the fat woman at the fair, on show to all." We overcame these difficulties.

In our men's ward were acute surgical cases, also acute pneumonia. Patients breathed their way back to, or out of this life. Patients with duodenal ulcers lived on milk, olive oil and kaolin and two hourly feeds, till they were as sick of the sight of them as we became of making them.

Men were admitted with peritonitis which in those days meant long weeks of careful nursing, dressings and weeks of anxiety for the poor wives and children.

We admitted patients for repair of hernias, which had to be nursed lying with only one pillow and a "donkey" under their knees. This I must explain, is a pillow with strong tapes which are meant to be tied to the top of the bed to stop the patient from slipping down the bed. These aids to comfort are now in disuse, as they are supposed to encourage thrombosis of the legs, and other disabilities.

These treatments were all in vogue, at the time, as the reign of antibiotics had not yet begun. It was four years away. M & B and penicillin, were only dreams in the minds of our scientists. I was taught to give rectal salines and a messy performance they often turned out to be. Even though these were given by the drip method, and had to be watched as a cat watches a mouse, the unfortunate patient often was in a damp bed. The only thing was, that if they had reached the state to need drip salines, they were in no position to worry too much.

The no-touch technique, was persistently drummed into us, as we were told that it was our fault if the patient were to develop any infection from our carelessness, so we lived in fear and trembling that someone's death would be at our doors and on our conscience for the rest of our lives.

To return to my first week on this ward, I was surprised to find that time went too quickly, and it was evening before I had had time to do half the things that were supposed to be crammed into those hours, on or off duty.

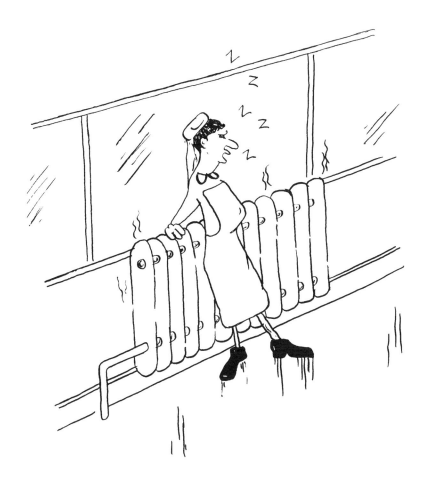

"Taking a break"

The pretty brown eyed, brown haired staff nurse, toiled one afternoon to show me the proper method of bathing a patient in bed. She taught me to put screens around the patient, who was a young man of thirty and recovering from dye poisoning. He was to be my guinea pig and could not have been enamoured of the prospect. Having obeyed her, I was then told to put his clean pyjamas on the radiator, place the towels ready, collect the bath blankets from the airing cupboard, fetch a bowl of hot water, methylated spirit and talcum powder for the "pressure parts." We then proceeded to strip the bed of the top blankets, covered him with a bath blanket and then rolled him from one side to the other, putting the other blanket under him.

I was told that on no account must any of his anatomy be exposed, except his face. Having washed this and dried, I coyly washed one arm then the other and returned them both to the fold. Both limbs, his back and front were treated in the same manner. His umbilicus was washed, his toenails cut and then he was given a flannel to wash his "nether parts," (all under the blankets.) This he modestly did, while we sternly gazed into space. This performance being over, I do not know who was the most exhausted, the patient, staff nurse or me. All concerned were duly thankful when this operation was over.

The first time I was addressed as "Nurse," I did not answer to it and when I realised that it was to me the title was given, I felt of much greater importance and a person entitled to respect at least.

Unlike the hospitals of today, we had no orderlies or S.E Nurses, and all the work not done by the Pro. was done by the maid of the ward.

Do not think this girl was a down-trodden personality, oh no. Hers was a life of ease and comfort, compared to ours. She was of medium height, with a good figure, slim and good shaped legs, which in her black silk stockings, she knew how to show off to advantage. Her dark hair was "permed", and when she had "changed" after lunch and the crockery was washed up, she emerged as a butterfly out of a chrysalis. With her feet encased in patent leather shoes, and her body enclosed in a tight fitting black dress, with pretty lace apron and pert cap perched on top of the "perm." She flirted and flounced her way around the ward, to the admiration of the men who were humming, to the then popular tune of "Tip toe through the tulips.," which she was always humming. I can never hear this tune without a feeling of nostalgia, for the first days of training, the days that are gone.

Christina came on duty in the morning and in time with her favourite tune she proceeded to sweep behind the beds which, after having been made, we pulled away from the wall. This done, we pushed them back to their proper abode. As she took her leisurely walk round the ward, she told the tale to the men, of her latest boyfriend: this fell on envious ears, for at that time we only had one evening a month (very soon to be altered by our Matron, who had only recently been appointed). She kept us in our place as she knew her rights, and as we seemed to have so few, we did not dare to retaliate.

At times, if her love affairs were going well, she would cut bread and butter for us, and if sister was off duty, would help us to take it round to the patients. At all times her eyes would gleam sharply at us, through her spectacles, as much to her disgust she was unable to do without them,

When I told Katie of our domestic help on our ward, she was envious, as their handmaiden was of a different calibre. She was oh so willing, but if they asked her to help them, she would plod off to do it, but was so slow that sister would wonder what she was doing and would come down like a ton of brick, for having taken her away from her appointed task. Apparently she also had a disconcerting habit of talking to herself, so that if by any chance one wandered into the kitchen, you would be greeted by Annie, "five, six, seven, now I must wash the cups, one, two, three cups, oh this one is not clean, there is the door bell, I must go and answer it. " Exit Annie.

Katie said that it nearly drove her mad. However, she looked very sane, as we sat in the evening, in our room eating apples, of which I am to this day very fond. Katie used to suck raw lemons, not because she liked them, but she had recently read in a magazine, that it was a total cure for acne. I had to give my considered opinion as to the merits of this method. I always told her that it was a great improvement, on the last treatment.

I should have named this book, "In Praise of Matrons." On looking back to those days, I felt somewhat sorry for our Matron. I don't suppose she needed my sympathy. She had only been appointed a little time before I arrived at the hospital, and must have had a great many old fashioned methods and prejudices to fight. What with committees, doctors and sisters all older. I think that she came to be well supported by many others, as they realised her calm good sense, and how she loved the work of this little ship, of which she was captain.

In appearance she was of medium height, slim and wore her plain navy dress with neat collar and cuffs with a certain amount of distinction. She had a thin face, with green twinkley eyes and a humourous twist to her mouth. She wore a large army cap, which seemed to suit her and her slim figure, and gave her added height. Her personality was such, that even to us, she was a good influence and as I can remember so much about her after all this time, it MUST have been good.

One of the traits of character, which endeared her to all of us, was her quirkish sense of humour. It would bubble forth at the most unlikely times. Witness the time when I was on night duty for the first time and had the lowest position, I was "runner." I helped all over the hospital wherever I was most needed. These duties included the job of cooking the midnight meals for the night sister and staff nurse. As I was initiated into these rites I was informed that their favourite dish was fried chips.

As potatoes were not always supplied to us, I had a brainwave. I searched the old fashioned kitchen and found "corn in Egypt," in the form of a large frying pan and a basin of dripping and loads of potatoes. The idea that I was trespassing and stealing never entered into my head. Cheerfully I set to and fried delicious crisp brown chips. Proudly I bore them to the sister and staff nurse. They ate them all and called for more. They were satisfied and my name was made.

In the morning, as I was going off duty, a figure appeared at the other end of the corridor, to my horror I recognised the cook. Her face was scarlet, her cap on one side, her wisps of hair flying, and to my even greater horror the frying pan full of congealed fat was in her hand. She was carrying it like a tennis racket. She sailed on down to the Matrons office, I did not wait to sail, I vanished.

Before I went off duty the next morning, I was told to report to the Matrons office. In fear and trembling I did so. "Did you use the frying pan leaving it filled with congealed fat?" "Yes Matron." "I do not remember giving out fat!" "No, Matron." "Well, in future, if you need anything extra, ask me for it, wash the utensils, and above all, DO NOT LET THE COOK KNOW, Good morning Nurse." Thankfully I went.

When I told Katie about this episode she went into fits of laughter and had to be revived by slapping her on the back. There was such a commotion going on in the nurse's home, that the assistant Matron wanted to know what it was all about. We did not enlighten her.

This silly episode was the subject of much jest, until it was supplanted by a much more ridiculous one. It concerned one, Maloney by name. She was sent on night duty as runner. She had the same duties to perform as I have already described to you. In appearance she was absolutely negative, had a soft South of Ireland voice and to quote the old adage, "she wouldn't say boo to a goose." (for my part I would not stay to say boo.)

She had been getting the meals and somehow she had a surfeits of fish to cook each night. Come the night there were herrings, with their gleaming bodies and their red eyes, denoting their health before they became entangled in the fishermens nets.

None of these perfections would comfort Maloney. She fried eggs (borrowed from the patients) with chips and pinned the offending herrings to the table, each little shining creature with its tail pierced by a drawing pin. There the cook found them in the cold light of morning. The rest I leave to your imagination.

In those days a Matron of a small hospital such as the William Garrett, had to be a Jack of all trades. She often had to deputise for the theatre sister. She took the part of a home sister, housekeeping sister. A great deal of the secretarial work was done by her and last but not least she even had to know something of radiography. I have never seen her anything else but calm and apparently untroubled. She certainly knew how to handle young head strong girls, such as we were at the time.

In order that the reader understands something of what comes after, I must explain that our hospital was affiliated to a larger and well know provincial hospital.

We took our state prelim, and our junior hospital exams, and if successful we passed on at the end of two years to the other one. Consequently we had a full four years training in all general work, particularly acute surgical. After this, we were turned out, complete with S.R.N and hospital badge, thinking we knew everything, only to find that we knew nothing and had to start to learn much that was not to be found in text books or hospital.

A few weeks after I arrived, I found that Katie Susan had a most amazing memory and could read a page of prose or poetry, and repeat it word for word without a mistake. More amazing still was the fact that at the thought of an exam she was petrified and later on when she took one, words failed her completely and the ink dried on the pen in sympathy. This trait of character was pertly the means of altering the whole course of her life. One of her talents was her gift of mimicry, this accomplishment nearly landed her in hot water and certainly did not add to her popularity with the person concerned.

Waiting for the sister tutor to arrive one morning, we became restive as she was a little late. Katie went out to the front of the lecture room, pulled Jimmy (the skeleton) from his cupboard. Then in a perfect imitation of Sister Marshal, she expounded the merits of Jimmy and she started to ask questions of the convulsed class. At the critical moment the door behind opened very quietly and there stood Sister Marshal. It was at that moment Katie was to be heard telling a delighted class "that's right nurse, you've got the idea but not quite" at the same time pointing out the winsome qualities of Jimmy's frame and personality.

CHAPTER 3

"Our Porter, Mr. King"

Sister Tutor was one of the prettiest and most dainty women I have met in hospital. Her age was about thirty, of medium height, a lovely figure, a heart shaped face, a milk and roses complexion and fair wavy hair. Her mouth was small and somewhat marred the beauty of her face by the peevish expression it gave to her. I do not think the casual eye would have noticed this, as in her navy dress, white apron, blue belt with silver buckle and her army cap on the back of her head, she was a picture. The navy knot seemed to accentuate the blue of her eyes.

In my own mind I always pictured her as being an orphan, brought up by two maiden aunts. These must have done their duty by her, educating her in early years at a small private school and later at a boarding school, from which she was taken suddenly as her aunts had by some mysterious means died. She then had to enter a cold cruel world and had chosen Nursing as the best of professions.

She had then met the MAN of her life, who was later killed in the war. Hence the rather perplexed expression on her otherwise perfect face. Many years later I heard the story of her life, till then and strange as it may seem, a lot of my imagining was not far wrong.

As a tutor she was painstaking and conscientious. She persevered with us and we passed our exams, to her pride and pleasure. I and a big bouncing vigorous girl from Wales had the doubtful honour of being the first two nurses from the William Garret to take the State Prelim and pass.

Sister Marshal was not only tutor but she was also responsible for the X-ray department.

The patients went in feeling curious, frightened or indifferent. Each reacting in a different way to his or her disposition.

All was warm and quiet as they entered. The patients were told to shed their garments, then given a kimono of pink or mauve sponge cloth. They were then asked to lie on the X-ray table and cover themselves with a blanket.

Then the sparks began to fly, lightening flashed from point to point, the patient became hotter and hotter, as sister moved knob after knob, first one then the another till she was satisfied. The X-ray was taken. By this time the patient was a mass of nerves and given permission, hastened to dress him or herself in the little cubicle reserved for the purpose. Exit patient in pursuit of the nearest lavatory.

At this time Georgy had been showing signs of restiveness. We knew that she was engaged to a soldier in the Guards and after a day off, she came back full of excitement. She and Nicholas had at last arranged to be married. This ceremony was to take place in two months time, at the farm in the Midlands from whence she came. She promptly gave in her notice and in the meanwhile we were regaled with the virtues, bravery and perfections of the "Obida" like lover. Later on when we were privilidged to meet this hero, we were all very disappointed. He was tall and solid looking but his conversation was absolutely unintelligible, partly owing to the fact that he made little sense, also he was a Geordie. However it was not necessary for us to understand him, as Georgy did all the translating. After the month had expired we never saw or heard anything of her again. Katie and I were feeling slightly more important, as it meant that we were gradually becoming more senior and could show off our ignorance to lesser fry.

One of the most important people in the hospital was our porter Mr. King, without him I do not think the institution could have carried on. In such a small place his duties were many.

He appeared in the morning, with a parcel of papers to sell to the patients. He toured the ward like a reigning monarch. Chatted with Christina as he dispensed his wares, listened to all the tales of "my operation," some new that morning and others he must have heard over and over again.

"Never mind dad, it'll all come out in the wash. Or, "It'll all be the same in a hundred years time." "Cheerio son, see you at the theatre, you and me will have the best seats." Thus cheering a young lad who had been in a nervous state, though we had tried to tell him that to have an appendix removed was not a very dreadful operation. King had achieved that which we could not.

In age he would have been about 40 years, he had been a sergeant in the Army and still walked as though he was still there. His handsome face delighted the eyes of the patients in the womens ward.

I found out later that he was a widower, also that his heart was set on Christina, but fickle jade that she was, she only appeared to flirt with him and tell him of her conquests. Just before I left the W.G., Christina had a shock, she heard that he was paying attention to a plump widow with a comfortable house and a nest egg. I do not think there was a lot of truth in it but after that rumour, Christina flirted openly no longer and the day was named and Christina faded out to the tune of wedding bells.

Not so King, he stayed on as porter and after I had finished my training, I visited the old place and there was King and he told me that he was a proud father of twins and Christina kept him in order and the twins in the same manner as she had us.

To us he was a treasure, "Send for King" he'll know what to do and he did. He was a tower of strength to a timid pro. as she made her way to the anaesthetic room with an equally timid patient, who was lying on the theatre trolley. "Cheer up dad, got y'r charts nurse?" when she arrived at the anaesthetic room, "Urry nurse, there's y'r gown and white boots over there, Old Whisky is giving the dope today and he likes his masks with an extra piece of gamgee". As the Pro. was supposed to help and wait on the anaesthetist, these tips were pearls of wisdom. He would then return to his own domain and leave the trembling Pro. to face "Old Whisky". By this time the patient would be told to "breathe deeply, that's right, breeaath deeeeply, again and again, thaats right!".

'Old Whisky', derived his name from the fact that he was a Scotsman and bore the name of a well known brand of spirits. Rumour had it that he was one of the firm. In appearance he was tall and thin, and non-descript looking and looked too tired to hold himself up.

At Christmas a party of artists came to give us a concert. There was a small band of minstrels and one of them gave a lively tap dance and sang to the tunes of "If you knew Susie as I knew Susie", also "Down in Nabasaki where the fellows chew tobaccy, and the women, whicky whacky whoo". We had the shock of our lives, this lively comedian was none other than "Old Whisky".

He was not really old but to our callow eyes he was a Rip Van Winkle. However our theatre sister, (who was also the assistant Matron), commonly known as Flossie Flannel Feet, had a great opinion of him and him of her. Her nickname was derived from her habit of walking with a soundless tread. This was not done on purpose to catch unwary Pro's, but she was naturally quiet and efficient in her normal life. She was tall and slim and short sighted and her bird like brown eyes peered at the world through a pair of thick lenses.

Later on when I came to know her, through having the coveted position of theatre Pro., I found her to be of a kind and humourous nature and dimly understood why "Old Whisky" was attracted to her.

Soon after I left, Old Whisky and Flossie were united in Holy Matrimony and from later news I think they were an ideal couple and a credit to the Nursing and Medical Profession.

Katie at this time had a great deal to contend with. The sister of the women's ward was not too popular with the Pro's, owing to her habit of expecting a harassed girl to do everything at the same time. She was not a good teacher, I think she took too much time telling the Pro all her mistakes and very seldom praising her good deeds. This sort of treatment was not of the kind that gave encouragement to the young nurses to proceed with their training.

I was fortunate in my first ward sister, but I found the first months of my training extra difficult. All that summer it was very hot and July and August passed in sweltering heat. I felt like an animal in a cage as I had been used to an outdoor life. My brothers and I, whatever part of the country we happened to be in, had walked, cycled, climbed and even swam in the sea or rivers. I missed them and they must have missed me.

Sometimes I felt and suffered in the same way as the old Texan who sang "Don't fence me in."

To overcome this I took to deliberately letting my mind wander on a magical journey, through a country where there were only cool fields, rocky coasts and sea as blue as the sky. In this world of fantasy I walked unaccompanied by the smell of lysol, there were no bedpans, soiled sheets to rinse, or sputum mugs to empty. No staff nurse to be heard saying "wake up, don't stand there dreaming, you'll never get that sluice done in time to go to your lecture!"

This habit of mine had some consequences, which did not prove fatal to anyone, but could have.

It was after I had been on the men's ward for two months that I was counted responsible enough to take charge of a small ward of convalescent patients, comprising of eight beds. These men were those who had had their sutures removed and were able to go to the toilet. At times we admitted patients who were in for investigation or for minor operations. In this ward I had the first experience of caring for an unconscious patient.

This man had been admitted the night before and had been taken to the theatre at about ten in the morning.

I had been taught the method of making an operation bed, so while the man (who had walked to the theatre) was away, I proceeded to do as I had been shown. All the bed clothes were turned back in such a manner to enable them to be removed en-masse, when the patient returned. The hot water bottles were in the bed, the locker was arrayed with a small towel, kidney dish, bowl of swabs, also a pair of tongue forceps with which we were supposed to save the patients life should he show signs of swallowing his tongue. As I prepared all these I fervently prayed that I should never have to use this instrument.

I had not long finished this preparation when the theatre trolley was heard and also what I took to be groans of agony. My friend King was there, joking with the staff nurse with what I thought to be undue levity. I hurried to remove the bedclothes as taught, helped them lift the man onto the bed and covered him over. She took his pulse, inspected my handiwork, showed me how to hold the kidney bowl under his chin and also how to hold the jaw forward to prevent him choking. Then with a swish of her apron and a last reminder to ring for help if I needed any and not to forget to record his pulse half hourly, till he was conscious, she turned and left the ward. When she had left, his groans grew louder and louder and the sweat poured from his forehead. I did not know which to do first, pull his chin forward, use the dreaded tongue forceps, or merely dash to the Matron and tell her that this was no profession for me.

However I did none of these things, as I was so sorry for him, with the tenderness of a mother for her first born child, I sponged his face with the swabs, stroked his fevered brow and held his hand, as he muttered unintelligible sounds. When eventually he had come round from the anaesthetic and staff nurse had inspected him, I then discovered that his only injury was a sprained ankle incurred as he played football. All that had been done to him was manipulation for adhesins.

If ever this man reads this book and recognises himself, he will now know that the little nurse who watched him, sweated as much or more than he did. To think of all the agony I had suffered on HIS account.

While I was in charge of this little ward, I took great pride in it and enjoyed keeping it in an immaculate state. One morning, having cleaned, polished, tidied the beds and arranged the flowers, to suit any martinet of a sister, I awaited her remarks with smug self satisfaction. She gazed all round the ward, ran her fingers along the ledges, looked at the straight line of top sheets and casters and apparently like Pilate of another year she could "find no fault". As I awaited the words of praise her eye fluttered to the clock, high up near to the ceiling."Nurse! did you dust the clock today?" "No sister." "Well do so now." With this, she stalked out. For once I was not only deflated, but speechless.

CALLING ALL SISTERS! BEWARE HOW AND WHAT YOU SAY, IT IS REMEMBERED LONG AFTER YOU ARE FORGOTTEN:

Katie was not getting along too well. According to the tale she told to me at night, her life was one long exercise! jumping in and out of hot water. On this particular day, nothing seemed to go right. The beds were not as they should be, she had given lemonade to Mrs. Jones, who was supposed be have milk, in all its various disguises.

In lecture Sister Marshal had been rather scathing on the subject of the figure-of-eight bandage, which Katie did not seem to be able to master very quickly and last but not least came the crowning indiscretion. As she was rather late back from lecture, she not only ran down the corridor (unheard of for a nurse) to the ward but as she reached the ward door, it opened, out came two men, one middle aged and the other young. To Sister Hawkins who was a stunned onlooker it appeared as though Katie had thrown herself into the arms of the young man and they both slipped on the highly polished floor. Both managed to regain their feet and with scarlet faces, took one look at each other in amazement. "Katie me darlin; what on earth are you doin' here"? "Percy!", in blank astonishment. By this time Katie had fled leaving Sister Hawkins in a state of great curiosity, agitation and mystification.

The explanation, according to Katie, was simple, it appeared that on the women's ward was a patient (PRIVATE) by the name of

Mrs. Pridefull. This lady was not popular with the nurses and I have a shrewd idea that it was only the well filled purse of her husband that was the attraction to the doctor concerned. After all a G.P. had to live. There was no National Health Scheme and the rich had to help to pay for the treatment given to the poor and the needy. It had its own rough justice. Mrs. Pridefull did NOT WANT to be well. What is more, she was going to have her money's worth from the hard earned money of her spouse. Her own doctor had treated her for everything he could, without surgery. Mrs. Pridefull had summoned the poor man from his rest and had convinced him that she was in agony. No! Never in the world of sickness was there such suffering; born with such fortitude. In self defence, it now being 2 a.m. the doctor had sent her in desperation to the hospital and called in the visiting surgeon Mr. Giles. He came accompanied by his nephew who was a student at one of the large teaching schools a few miles away.

To return to the entrance of Katie, in such a dramatic manner, Mrs. Pridefull had been duly satisfied that she was getting the best of attention, Mr. Giles and Percy O'Brien, were preparing to go and find a suitable method of restoring their lost vigour due to the masterful Mrs. Pridefull and her overbearing manner.

As his name might tell you, Percy O'Brien hailed from Ireland and by coincidence he lived not far from Katie's ancestral home. In days gone by he, Katie and her sisters had danced the light fantastic at the local hops. She knew he was in London but in her casual manner had forgotten which hospital was honoured by his presence. Also she had not seen necessary to inform him that she was at a hospital where men in the medics profession never looked any lower than at a sister or higher than the Matron, so you can well imagine that our scope was limited.

As we were told not to become familiar with the patients, it was a sterile kind of existence, not conducive to an easy courtship. Some of the nurses like Nurse Prim were defeated at the start and I feel sure they are now disenjoying the fruits of celibacy.

This incident did nothing to improve Katie's popularity, I am sure Sister Hawkins only wished it had been she who had been called "darlin", in that lifting Irish voice.

Next morning Katie had a letter from Percy asking if it was permissible to take a fellow countrywoman to a dinner and dance, at the EARLIEST opportunity.

This was accepted with great alacrity. Like all of us, even though well fed, we seemed to be eternally hungry. Katie was no exception. She was doomed from that day. She was never able to put S.R.N. after her name but was a great help to Percy in a busy rural practice. She was used to this life, so it was not a hardship to her. But this was then all in the future.

SHE DID NOT TELL ME TILL MUCH LATER, THAT HE HAD ALWAYS BEEN HER HERO.

CHAPTER 4

"Enter, Nurse Rochester"

To return to my own trials and meagre triumphs. More of the first than the last, as a rule. This being one of those rare exceptions.

It was a Sunday afternoon, only Sister Fletcher and I were on duty, she was sitting in the ward at her desk, keeping her eye on the visitors who had streamed in at two o'clock. Two were allowed at the bedside, at times more would enter and hang around the bedside of those without any. When she was there, they had little or no success.

Worried wives or children would enquire if "dad would soon be'ome, as our boy in the Navy is comin' on leave and we'd like to 'ave a celebration of both events".

She did her best to comfort the anxious and help the helpless. Many faces left the ward looking brighter for having been reassured by her. Others (not many), were sad and drawn looking as she had had to break the news, that a beloved son or father, would never see their home again.

I was in the kitchen cutting bread and butter for the patient's tea and looking forward to mine when suddenly the phone rang, sister answered it, I heard her saying "in a half an hour? yes I'll have him ready". As I was the only other nurse on the ward, she came to me and spoke to me as an equal and not as to a J.P. of only a few weeks standing. "There is a patient being admitted soon, he has to be prepared for an operation, for acute appendicectomy. The theatre sister is off duty and I shall have to take the patient down to the theatre, I have to rely on you to make the operation bed as you have been taught and also to give the patients their tea, do the B.P. round and start to wash them, by which time the other nurses should be back from their off duty. Do you think you can manage it?". "Oh! yes sister", I cried in enthusiasm. "You can trust me".

The patient was admitted and although there was much work and little time to do it all in, she took me with her to show me the technique of preparation. She gave the man (who turned out to be young and handsome, aged twenty four) an injection of atropine, this helps to dry up the secretions from the mucous membranes and stops the patient choking under the general anaesthetic.

I was very sorry for him, as he appeared to be in great pain and his knee was drawn up to his abdomen, this she explained to me, was a great help in the diagnosis as it was one of the signs of the condition. As for me, well, I was very frightened for him as it looked so grotesque.

She soon had him ready and our friend King with his usual cheery manner was on the scene, accompanied by the theatre trolley. We all lifted him on to this and they departed leaving me alone to carry out her instructions. It was not a great thing to have to do but to me at the time it was of terrific importance.

I managed it all, even to get King to have the electric blanket ready and everything in order by the time he returned.

Sister Fletcher took one look around the ward; her eye missing nothing. Her face slowly broke into a smile. "You have done well nurse." No more, but it was enough to make me feel as though I was a REAL NURSE.

This blissful attitude was soon dispelled, when a few days later, she discovered some stale bread which had been put into the dustbin, instead of the big-bin which was kept outside the kitchen door. "I thought you were going to make a good nurse but now I am forced to change my opinion of you". Exit my halo and wings, I was very deflated.

Some weeks before I left this ward, our Irish staff nurse was transferred to the women's ward and in her stead came one of the best nurses I have met, Nurse Rochester. Many years later I was to see her name in the national newspaper. This was after the second war, she was being presented with a medal for devotion to duty and bravery. She had carried on in the theatre, during one of the most heavy raids of the war. There was much else to the story, I could well imagine her in any emergency as one of the most cool.

At the time of which I write, she was small and had a good figure. Here eyes were large and almost black. Her skin was olive coloured, her hair black and even then, was streaked with grey. At all times she moved quickly and quietly, her expression full of lively intelligence. To most of us she seemed to be an enigma, her age, we never knew. She appeared to have no other life but the hospital. On her days off she was known to visit some relative in the home counties. Her one great hobby was reading, she also had a large collection of ebony ornaments. Where she had bought these none of us knew.

As a nurse her worth could not be assessed. As a teacher there were non to excel. She had the power to impart her knowledge to the most dull and even the simplest method of treatment became interesting. She was exacting and nothing but perfection was good enough for her. To the patients she was kindness itself. Nothing was too much for her to do, as long as it was for their good. She drilled into us the idea that we should not be ashamed to do anything, however trivial. As she practiced what she preached, we had no argument. I have tried to live up to this ideal but I am afraid, that like many other, I have fallen by the wayside.

It was she who taught me that NONE are indispensable. One day, as we were making beds together, she remarked that her holidays were very soon due. In a spasm of hero worship I said "Oh! what shall we do without you?" She turned to me and said, "No one is indispensable but some are more missed than others". Young as I was I never forgot this maxim.

I shall always remember the morning when the phone rang and we were told that a patient was to be admitted at once. The harassed G.P. had diagnosed him with pneumonia. The ambulance arrived and the patient was brought in and put to bed with the usual paraphernalia for the patient who suffered from this condition. He was dressed in a gamgee jacket and his pillows were built up, to enable him to breath more easily. His history was taken from his relatives and the screens were left around him, ready for the visiting physician.

As I left him, after tidying his locker and straightening it, I turned and looked at him and to my amazement his face appeared to be grinning in a most horrifying manner and he seemed to be in some kind of spasm. I ran (yes, I defied all rules against such a procedure) for Nurse Rochester, she came, took one look at the patient, pulled the screens together, told me not to leave him and went to the room where the dressing trolleys were kept. She came back almost immediately and on the trolley were instruments which to me at the time were a mystery. There were syringes, test tubes and a phial of some substance, well know to the troops at the later part of the Great War. This was merely marked A.T.S. (Anti Tetanus Serum). At that moment the G.P. appeared, took one look at the patient, glanced at the trolley, went out and scrubbed up. When he came back he injected the serum and did a lumber puncture, then immediately after went to the phone, rang the local isolation hospital and in ten minutes this poor man was on his way there.

She then told me, that as soon as she had seen the expression on his face she had known what was the matter and by having everything ready, she had anticipated the doctor's requirements and so had saved valuable time. She explained that his grimace was know as the "sardonic grin" and is peculiar to the patient suffering from tetanus. In later lectures we were told that it is the "most terrible disease that mankind can suffer from". The germ attacks the muscles and at the slightest movement or sound, they contract into terrible spasms. The horrifying part of this disease, is that the patient is conscious all of the time. I am sorry to say, that this man of only twenty four, did not recover and this tale has not a happy ending. He died a few days later and he had been kept under anaesthetic as much as possible as this is the only way to relieve the pain of the muscle contraction.

When we were off duty, most of us felt too tired to go places, but thanks to Sister Marshal, we did eventually find that if we went out we felt much more alive. As our off duty in the first year was restricted, we could not make many plans except for our days off. In the evening of the day before our day off we were allowed a late pass until twelve o'clock, or as it was called, a theatre pass. We could have a sleeping out pass if we were in a position to satisfy the Matron that we had relatives or friends to stay with.

We always had to present ourselves at the office at nine in the morning, complete with clean apron and cuffs. We were never supposed to be seen outside the ward without these talisman. I used to thing that should we do so, we would be pounced on by an ogre from the dark corners of the corridors, stuffed inside a bag and be heard of no more.

On my first day off, I felt like a bird on the wing. It was a lovely day, I had my breakfast in bed, this being allowed, if we notified the housekeeping sister (also theatre sister). It seemed the height of luxury, then I had a long session in the bath, as the nurses home was singularly empty, I had not anything particular to do until after lunch, for which I proposed to partake at Lyons Corner House, this being the height of my ambition and finances. After this I had made plans to visit friends of my school days. They lived about three miles from the W.G. I was quite excited as I had not seen them for some time.

Mr. and Mrs. Chandler received me as though I had only seen them a day or so ago, Jill and Sam, were due home at tea time. They all wanted to know about this profession called nursing. I think they thought I could have had a much easier life, as a shorthand typist or, ANYTHING but this. However, after tea, we made use of my theatre pass and went to a play and to supper afterwards. Despite their disapproval of my choice of work, they cordially invited me to get a sleeping out pass and spend my next day off with them. This I decided to do. It seemed wonderful to be away from the atmosphere of the hospital and have a little of home life, even if only for a few hours.

Many times during the next two years, I was tempted to leave, as the hours were long and it was hard to think that other girls and their boy friends could make plans to go out on Saturday afternoons and Sundays while we were tied to the sluice and the bedpans.

These kindly people never knew how much I had them to thank, for the fact that I eventually made the grade. But to return to that first day off. I just managed to reach the hospital in time to meet the night sister who gave the key of the nurses home to her runner. With this she opened the front door made me sign the late pass book, locked it and returned to the patients.

Katie was waiting for me and wanted to know all the news of the outside world and was only waiting for her next evening with Percy. As she had hers first, it seemed a long time to wait until the next piece of freedom. He was a great deal irritated at the way we were treated like school children and yet, at the same time, were expected to do the work of two women and had only the rights of the mentally retarded. These were not my words but they were very near the truth. As I have said before, our Matron did her best to alter these rules and in time did.

Although we had only been a month in the hospital, we felt as though we had gone through a life time.

We had to make our own amusements and one day we were treated to a good laugh.

There were two Welsh girls, one of whom I have already mentioned, here name was Mary Ellen Price. Tall, curvaceous, tawny hair, bright green eyes and a high colour. She was noisily cheerful and had a lovely clear soprano voice. Her friend, who answered to the name of Gwyneth Jones was dark, plump and also cheerful and her black eyes snapped and sparkled and at every opportunity she laughed, wheezed and choked. She was a prime favourite with the patients. Her voice was a heavenly contralto and at times when Mary and Gwyneth were in the nurses home, they would have a duet and their pet tune was the old hymn "Aberystwith". At times we thought it lovely but when we wanted to study or sleep at nights, this Eistedford was not so popular and distinctly, not received in the spirit that such sacred music should have been.

This afternoon Mary and Gwyneth were off duty together, Katie and I were trying to study a little, suddenly there was a burst of melody from the bathroom on our floor. We were at a loss to understand why they were in there together. Their voices rang out, ranging from their favourite, "Abide with Me", "Eternal Father", and of course "Land of My Fathers", all these sung in the Welsh language. After an hour, the singing died down and we went to ask if anything was the matter and why were they so long in there. We were callously told to go and "boil ourselves". This was not very helpful, as we could not even get into the bath to do so, so we went.

Teatime passed and there was no sign of Mary or Gwyneth and at supper we heard the whole tale.

It was fashionable at the time to be sunburnt. The more oriental one could look, the better. Most of us use to retire to the local Lido and disport ourselves to the fickle light of the sun. The two Welsh girls had not that type of skin to respond to such treatment and the results were blisters and peeling skin.

They then had a bright idea. Having read in one of the women's magazines that if permanganate of potash was diluted with water and the skin painted therewith the results would be as good as if not better than the real thing. They had a much better scheme. They made a home made Riviera by filling the bath with a solution of the magic liquid. Then sat on the side of the bath with their legs immersed. To while away the time they sang, as I already told. After an hour, when they thought their legs were sufficiently bronzed, the water was let out, (this explained the dead silence) dried them and turned to the bath. To their horror, it was dyed the colour that they had hoped to be. It was a warm attractive brown. Having grasped the situation, the next thing to do was to rectify it, before anyone in authority saw it.

The maid the next morning was heard to be complaining that her "Vim" had all gone, she did not know where, We did!

Katie and I took our pleasures differently, we were fond of devouring peach melba at the haven of the poor "Lyons". One morning when we were off duty together, and having devoured our usual, we were still hungry, so we gazed into the window of a pastrycooks and finally went in and settled for doughnuts, freshly baked, rolled in sugar and dripping raspberry jam. Our upbringing and fear of being recognised by anyone from the W.G. made us refrain from eating them in the street, so we made our way to the Roman Catholic Church. Katie led me to one of the seats and having geneflected on the way, we then knelt down and with our heads bowed, ate the succulent delicacies.

The old priest looked at us with a very puzzled expression on his tired face. I think if he had known what we were doing, he would not have minded at all. I cannot explain it, but we were always hungry. It was not because we were not fed well, as we counted ourselves lucky, the Matron did not believe in cutting expenses at the cost to the nurses health. This was and still is a false economy practiced in many hospitals.

Having fortified ourselves in this manner, we returned to duty, to meet any serious emergency that would arise.

As it was visiting afternoon, the job that was waiting for me, was the laundry. To a later generation or even a Pro. in a larger hospital, this will not mean much.

We had no laundry on the premises and an outside firm had the contract. Large baskets of laundry came back every Friday. The care taken by this firm to please, would make the modern nurse envious. Every article was returned wrapped in blue tissue paper. They were snow-white and had just the right amount of starch. The aprons were crisp and shining, caps, collars and cuffs, just right.

The other side of the picture was different. All this beautiful linen and all the bed linen on the ward had also to be sorted, counted and re-checked, out and in. As I was at that time a J.P. it was my work to retire to the sluice room, shut the door, separate each kind of article, put it with its fellow, count them, record it and send for staff nurse or sister to check and put them in the baskets left by the firm.

I did not mind this "extra work", as I used to retreat to my dream world. It was even worth having to count them all over again and being ticked off for having miscounted.

The worst part of this job was that before any soiled article was sent out, it was the Pro's work to rinse every stain out of them. I can assure you that this was not an enviable task. To make it more unpleasant, we had only common soda and soap to use and as a disinfectant we used Lysol. Our hands in the first year, were not those of nurses in popular novels. cooling and soothing to the fevered brow.

Do not think that we only did these chores, they were intercepted with more interesting work. We were first allowed to look with rapt attention, while some hallowed being, e.g. staff nurse or sister, did a dressing, poultice, enema, hot pack, hypodermic or intramuscular injection. Having been shown how, we were then allowed to lay up the trolley or tray, then later were made to do the treatment under supervision and later still we had to do it on our own and have it inspected by the one in charge at the time. Keeping up with practical nursing, lectures by sister tutor, forcing ourselves to go out on our off times to acquire fresh air and exercise (as advised by those who had once been in the same position as us) and trying to squeeze a little private and social life, was not easy and took a lot out of us, physically and mentally. Also we were still young and emotionally insecure and unstable.

Looking back to it, I think I would not have it any different.

CHAPTER 5

"Doctors May, Nurses Never"

After about three and a half months, I was transferred to the womens ward. Katie was sent to the men's ward. I felt envious of her and said a last goodbye to the men and in my heart I was sorry to be leaving the protecting mantle of Sister Fletcher's influence and more sorry to have to leave for the first time the most wonderful Staff Nurse Rochester, but still I had to and to this day, her teachings still bear fruit.

This move was not my choice. I did not like it at all. I have already spoken of Sister Hawkins as described by hearsay and was prepared to hate her on sight.

However when I came to know her a little better, I found that she was a woman of strong religious views and in her own way was a conscientious nurse. She never could be called a loveable woman. She was always in a hurry (or so appeared to be) and if annoyed, or worried, her face would flush to an unbecoming red and her rather protruding pale blue eyes seemed to stick out all the more. I did not at the time recognise the condition it portrayed, I think she must have been the victim of an enlarged thyroid gland and that accounted for the flap that she used to get in at the slightest opportunity.

She was easily aerated and I seemed to find myself in continuous hot water. Luckily the pretty Irish staff nurse was there to temper things down a little.

At first, I thought that the women on the ward were a miserable lot. After I had been there only a few days, I discovered that they were nearly all of them, most grateful for all that was done for them. To many, it was the first rest that they had had in all their lives, especially those who were married and had a family.

They were also very good at hiding sins from Sister Hawkins and if they were allowed up, would always lend a helping hand to raw recruits like me.

One of them would whisper to me, "Sister likes it this way nurse" or "I'll clear the bowls away after she is gone to tea". I would return from my own tea to find bowls, tooth mugs and flowers removed for the night, so that we could carry on and make the beds. These we were supposed to make, if empty, in two minutes. The occupied ones in three. No time or consideration was given to the fact that often a patient would ask for a bedpan, or upset a tumbler of water over the clothes, or even take that moment to vomit all over the clean sheets that you might have just put on.

I also discovered that as women have different organs to their bodies, this makes for more complications.

25

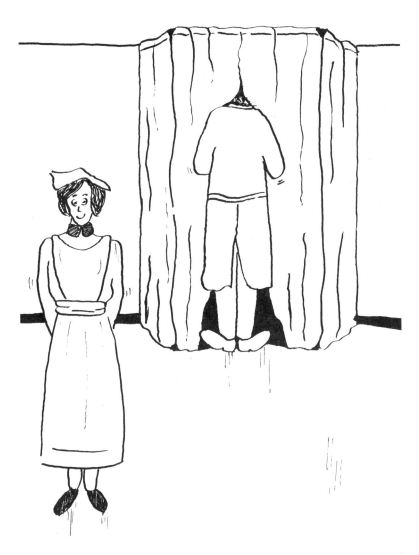

"Doctor on the job"

By this time, I was to be trusted to do simple treatments, such as taking temperatures, simple enemas, hot fomentations etc. I had been promoted to the rank of Pro. instead of J.P. This meant that I dusted the right side of the ward in the mornings instead of the left and had the doubtful privilidge of having the door held open for me by the newest addition to our training school. This shrinking violet, was a damsel from the wilds of the Yorkshire Moors. Her father owned many acres, had plenty of BRASS, but according to Jane Brodie, did not like parting with it. So she decided to take up this profession, to escape tyranny and personal poverty. Evidently pop had played holy Hamlet but as his daughter was as stubborn as he, they came to no other conclusion. Jane had her own way. With her direct nature and the strength and courage of herYorkshire forbears, she carved a name for herself, at a later date.

To return to me, I had an old lady to nurse at that time, almost had to special her, I think because no-one else relished the case. Of course I had no alternative. She was eighty years old and suffered from that most awful complaint, Parkinson's Disease (shaking palsy). The old woman Mrs. Fairhurst had to be washed, fed and treated like an elderly baby and not a very attractive baby at that.

It was difficult to imagine her as a child or even a blushing bride. However one day when her daughter was there she started to tell me that her mother lived with her and she found it increasingly difficult to look after her. So the doctor had sent Mrs. Fairhurst to us, to give her a rest. Then to my absolute astonishment she told me that her mother had been a chorus girl at a well known variety hall. All this was hard to believe but I gazed at the old lady with renewed interest and dimly felt sorry for her without the slightest understanding.

One thing I could well get used to was the sight of Mrs. Fairhurst asleep. She had some ill fitting false teeth and these clattered together like castanets when she was awake, but when she was asleep they looked most macabre as they were nearly falling out, but never quite did, most disconcerting.

I have not mentioned much of the doctors, as these illustrious beings were far removed from the world of sluice rooms, laundry, lectures and toilets.

We were taught **"Doctors may make mistakes, but nurses never"**. "Ours is not to reason why, ours but to do or die." Therefore, when the great being did his round, all we did was to obey their orders as relayed to us by the sister or staff nurse.

Even though we had no time or opportunity for dalliance or interest in them, the women patients had.

At the time of which I write, there were two patients of diverse personalities and complaints. They had only one thing in common, their passionate devotion to their own G.P. and their jealousy of each other.

Mrs. Cherub was far removed from her name, she was young (about thirty years) and weighed nineteen stone. Her face was the only part of her to match her name. It was round, pink and pleasant looking. Her hair was long, wavy, fine and flaxen. She had come to us to be stabilised as to her diet. Her weight was such, that young as she was, it was difficult to do the ordinary household duties.

In the bed opposite to her was Mrs. Haggis. Now Mrs. Haggis was a different proposition. She was dark, sallow and slim. The uncharitable would say "skinny".

In age she was fifty. I think she gave her age to us as forty. Thanks to the doctor, we knew differently. She had come in for an investigation, with a view to an operation on her gall bladder. Her hair was so lank and scraggy looking that she kept it hidden under a "boudoir cap". The effect of her beady little black eyes peeping out from under a fringe of lace, has to be seen to be believed. It gave her the appearance of a well dressed monkey. When she was annoyed, they snapped viciously. Mrs. Cherub, seemed to be the chief cause of this.

Their doctor, a pleasant cheerful man, who in private life had a lovely looking wife and a noisy brood of handsome children, treated them impartially and kindly. I do not think he knew the havoc he created in those women's hearts and the bitter dislike that they held for each other.

All the other women used to wait for this entertainment. On the great morning, Mrs. Cherub, would proceed to comb and brush her hair, like a mermaid. This she did with a smug expression on her face, never even glancing at the other side of the ward. Already she would have put on a spotless nighty, with embroidery and threaded with pink ribbon. When these adornments were complete, she would then sit up without moving until the doctor had done his round. She looked just like a child dressed up for a party and had been told by her parent not to move.

On the other side of the ward, the more sophisticated Mrs. Haggis also waited. her ensemble was quite different. She wore a fetching creation of deep mauve. It consisted of a nightdress, bed jacket and boudoir cap, all trimmed with coffee coloured lace. With her sallow coloured skin, this did not invite much admiration. When the unsuspecting man had disappeared and sister had gone to lunch, they would start. What the man had said, "to which and what and to whom".

Mrs. Cherub would laugh and wheezed till she shook like a jelly but not so Mrs. Haggis. To her it was deadly serious, she neither smiled nor did she laugh.

Later on, Mrs. Cherub went home to a devoted family, her weight reduced considerably. I do not know for how long, as she confided in me, that she was fond of fish and chips, cakes and all the things which to her made life more interesting but were not "what the doctor ordered".

Mrs. Haggis, had her operation and when they had examined her they found that, which, did not make for a long stay on this earth. She was sent home when her stitches were removed, to be looked after by her husband and daughter.

If only she had gone to the doctor who she adored, when she first noticed her symptoms, perhaps, who knows, she might have lived till a greater age. However she did not. Ever after, I always felt a certain guilt; that I did not care much for her as a person, but still, she never knew.

Her husband collected her with a taxi and very unobtrusively presented us with a large box of chocolates, which we ate as usual, with great gusto.

It was at this time that my dangerous habit of day dreaming led me into hot water as usual.

One evening, when most of the routine work had been done, staff nurse called me to her and told me to put the screens around Mrs. Shepard, the old lady in the corner who had been very ill, but was now, much better. 'Granny', as we called her, had had bronchitis and her doctor who was nearly as old as she and very old fashioned in his methods, had ordered leeches to be applied to her skinny chest. This had been done and had been removed when they were repleted by the simple method of putting salt on them. The affected area had to be painted with iodine. I was asked to do this easy treatment. You would not conceive that anyone could get into trouble doing this, but I did.

I put the screens around her, having laid the tray in the approved style. I then proceeded to disrobe Granny Shepard. I relieved her of her nightdress and gamgee jacket and started painting. First I applied a postage stamp to the front of her chest. I vaguely thought that it looked odd, so I painted one on the back. This did not satisfy me, it looked unsymmetrical, so I dreamily went on with my artistic efforts until I had painted an iodine vest, complete with armholes merging into shoulder straps, as sold in the shops as vests with "built up tops".

I then called staff nurse to inspect my handiwork and awaited her words of appreciation. These never came, her pretty face flushed with anger and she nearly choked with wrath. "You will report to sister in the morning". There was not much for her to say, but she said it very well.

At nine in the morning I duly presented myself at Sister Hawkins desk. "Put the screens around Mrs. Shepard's bed and I will come and see the damage". In fear and trembling, I did so. When sister came, I removed the clothing and to my absolute stupification, there was NO IODINE VEST. Sister looked at me as though I was mentally deficient, as indeed I felt.

There was nothing for her to say, so I thankfully removed the screens.

I sought the explanation of this phenomenon and had it explained that iodine disappears if the patient perspires, this Mrs. Shepard obligingly had done!

Soon after this episode, one of the junior night nurses went off sick. This was rectified by taking me, then a Pro. of about five months standing and raising my status, by appointing me to be night runner. The nurse selected for this honour, was as the name implies, "a runner". This was literally true, the nurses duty was to help in a junior capacity, in all the wards, at appointed times. Usually she followed a written time table.

She was responsible for the meals of night sister and staff nurse, sluicing all soiled linen in the children's ward and also relieved "nights off". As we at the time only had one night a month, this was not too often. All this was counted to be good experience. As I had no ambition to be a laundress, I did not agree.

I was on duty all the morning; and after dinner I was told to go to bed in the vain hope of being able to sleep. For more reasons than one, this was impossible. I was excited and apprehensive at the same time.

After being called at seven thirty, I had a bath to see if I could freshen myself. As I was new to this duty I was very early to the dining room. This had an unfamiliar look, as though there had been a wedding party and all the guests had departed, leaving their empty chairs and something of their perfume and ghostly personalities.

Presently the nurses arrived and dispelled this illusion. I felt that I should never get used to eating herrings and marmalade at that unnatural hour. After a few times, I forgot to comment on it.

As I was attempting to eat, the night sister arrived. She was a small, plump, round faced bustling Welsh woman of about thirty five years. Her hair was sovereign in colour, her skin rosy. Owing to her Celtic origin, her voice had the sing song lift to it. When excited, her voice rose to a crescendo.

Later on, I discovered that her habit was to "do her round" at two o'clock, dressed in a navy cloak,lined with scarlet. In her hand, she carried a torch, with a very bright light.

By this time, the nurse on the ward would be congratulating herself that at last, the ill patient in the first bed was in a fitful slumber and at last she could sit down and sew the pile of gamgee jackets or the many tailed bandages, left by the day sister, in case the nurse had a few idle moments before four a.m.

Sister Evans would announce her presence by a swish of starched clothing and of course, THE TORCH.

Having catechised the nurse on the patients welfare she then started, with her satellite tagging on after her. Beginning with number one ill patient she shone the bright light on to him, to see if he was alive AND sleeping. By this time the person concerned was wide awake. She then passed on to her next victims.

After she had gone to the other wards the Pro. would then seek to repair the damage done by this cyclone. Once more she would have to dole out a bedpan or a cup of Ovaltine, then perhaps, with luck, the chores might be done in time to satisfy the day sister.

This went on without interruption until one man who had a fractured skull and multiple injuries (but was on the road to recovery) was awakened in a like manner. As this was not the first time his blood pressure had rose and into the delighted ears of all the other sufferers, now wide awake, there fell the words like music "What the blank, blank, blank - - - - are you doing, waking me up when I have just fallen asleep. Blank blank and a lot more of this type of language. The man had said that which the nurse and others had long wanted to say and had not the courage. Apart from this idiosincracy, she was a good and kind night sister.

When I had finished breakfast, on my first introduction of this owl-like existence, I was told to look at the time table which was prepared for the 'runner'. Having digested these words of wisdom, I proceeded along the corridor, to the men's ward, feeling as though I had grown several inches taller. No nurse could be bolder, with my cloak around my shoulders and a small case in my hand (this only contained a book and a lecture book) I felt that at last I was a NURSE. Not the one who had come to the W.G. HOS-PITAL but the one who graces the front cover of all the magazines.

This was dispelled as soon as I reached for a sputum mug and I found that I still had to climb on a chair.

I had looked forward to seeing the men's ward again, but as some months had elapsed since I first entered it I hardly recognised it. In fact, the whole of the hospital held a totally unfamiliar and unreal appearance. I think when the dawn at last came, it was still more bleak and cold looking.

It was eight forty five when we reported on to the wards. From then on, I was told to do the round of bottles and bed pans. In the meanwhile the nurse of the ward, took the report from the day sister, took the charts from the beds, took temps and did any four hourly treatment. Having in the odd minutes, collected the eggs from the patients and marked each with his name, (they had to provide their own for breakfast) and given drinks to any who wanted one, I then helped nurse "do backs" and then make all the patients comfortable.

After this, she then put the charts, (with written up drugs) for the night sister to check.

At a later hour I went to the womens ward, and cut stacks of bread and butter and put it in the pantry, ready for the morning.

As I have already mentioned, I had to get the meals ready for the night sister and staff nurse, my own and proceed to the children's Ward and wash nappies and hang them in the drying room which was attached to that ward. If any unfortunate Pro. did not happen to carry out this chore in a manner satisfactory to the day sister, she was called back, after her morning meal, to rectify her erring ways.

In the morning, I had to help the staff nurse wash the babies and little children. Although I was the elder of a large family, I was still terrified to touch them, they felt so small and delicate. Later on I was to think they had a natural resistance and were made of India rubber.

CHAPTER 6

"In Memory Of Mr. Thin"

Having survived this strange night, I managed to get off duty without being "sent for". I was going to bed, but I found home sister waiting for me. I had to move my things over to the night nurses home. After I had managed this, I found Katie waiting for me. Would I come with her to partake of light refreshment, I did. At the same time I had to hear of her troubles. All was not well with her and Sister Fletcher, they did not appear to see eye to eye.

Also her love affairs were not all that could be desired. Percy, never a very patient man at the best of times, was trying to persuade her to forsake the W.G. and go back to the Emerald Isle and marry him, after he had a years experience. Katie was equally determined that she would not return yet, as I think she felt too young to shoulder such a responsibility. Percy had his moods and fancies, his persuasive ways and his devastating temper, which his patients in Ireland were to talk of and make a subject for conversation, at their various meetings of any kind. Although he was only a young man and brilliant, he looked, even at this early age, like a professor.

He would walk in a quick and jerky manner, his hands swinging in an ungainly way. His deepset blue eyes would peer from a long mass of brown hair, which was in a constant state of disrepair. He was like a lot of others, generous and mean in turns. All these things made Katie who knew and loved him, to be a little cautious.

Having devoured an ice cream and various other luxuries, we then wended our way back to the hospital, she to the men's ward and I to have a bath and try and be in bed as the rule said, by half past twelve. You would think that it was easy to sleep after being up a night and till that time. At first it seemed so strange, but we were very soon used to it. I have never liked night duty, I always felt as though I was missing so much of life. I had a tendency to think and feel like Perephone. Many of my friends then and later, did not agree with me and took posts as night sisters and seemed to thrive on it!

This, my first period of night duty, was meant to last only three months, which at that time, was considered to be the usual, but somehow it stretched out to five months.

One night I was relieving on the men's ward, as it was the Pro's night off. I came on duty and took the report from the day sister. There had been a new admission. He was a man of forty years old and he was diagnosed to be suffering from haematemesis (vomiting blood from the stomach). If I had been more senior, I would have understood more about it. Now, if a patient should be unfortunate enough to be brought in with such an unpleasant complaint, he would be treated with blood transfusions and unless the cause was hopeless at the start he would be returned to the bosom of his family having had the appropriate treatment or operation.

To return to this night, which to me, as a very junior Pro. was one I shall never forget. We were taught that the responsibility was not ours, that there was always a trained sister to call in and hers was the responsibility. We were unimpressed with these words, as we felt loaded with care.

After I had taken the report from the day sister, I did a round to say good evening to the men and also to collect the charts. Having done this, I looked down the ward in acute dismay. In the first bed on the right, there was a very ill man. At the side of his bed was an aweinspiring sight. It was a bottle hanging from a hook on a stand. Attached to it was a length of tubing and glass connections, which disappeared mysteriously under the bedclothes. I had been shown how and what to do with this apparatus, which was known as a drip saline. This was introduced into the body via the rectum, an exceedingly messy business, for patient and nurse. It was a tricky job at the best of times to make this elusive catheter stay in place but when the patient was a man who was bleeding internally, vomiting and in the throes of delirium, well! the task was well nigh impossible. He was only allowed to have ice to suck and as he had a raging thirst, it was a case to daunt the stoutest heart, even had I been many years older and much more experienced.

I cast my eye farther down the ward. There was a man with peritonitis, he was on four hourly hot fomentations and injections and had only recently come off the danger list. Passing to the end of the ward, was an old man Jimmy, he was a gentleman of the road and to his acute embarrassment, had been brought in with a strangulated hernia. He had been at the casualty ward of the local institution, (still known as the "work' us") when he was "took bad" and he had been horrified to think that all his "body heat" had gone down the sink. He had been washed and shaved in more parts of his body than he had seen for years. After he had recovered from the anaesthetic, the nurses had the utmost difficulty in persuading him that he had to stay in bed. I was told that he would get up in his hospital shirt and wander around looking for the front door. He was always afraid that someone would pinch his money, that he said he had hidden in a hedge row, outside the casualty ward.

On the other side were just the ordinary cases, except at the farther end where there was an old man with what we call cardiac oedema (dropsy). He was the first and last person I ever saw to be treated by the insertion of little silver tubes, each with small holes in them,(Southey Tubes). As the old man was so grossly swollen, his feet were put in a bath and the water drained therein. It was irrigated with what was known as Carol Dakin's Solution.

This man was ill and needed a lot of attention. His face was red and shining and his fiery blue eyes looked out at us with frustration and despair. He could hardly do anything for himself and how he resented it. The last one who passes through my minds eye, is Mr. D. Dyer, who was an inoffensive little man. He had a sallow skin, kind apologetic eyes that reminded one of a dog. He only had a simple hernia and was no trouble during the day, he spoke in an American nasal tone with a north London accent.

At night, this little fellow was no longer harmless, he became a menace. HE SNORED. It was no ordinary snore. It started as a Zephyr whispering through a cornfield on a summers day. It gradually increased in volume, till it became the sound of a trumpet and rose to a crescendo and then suddenly there was blessed silence. The other men would hold their breath with him. Would it stop, or not, No! there was a terrible snort and then the process would start all over again. I tried all methods to stop him during the time I was on that ward, all to no avail.

To return to that night, at ten o'clock the night sister came and checked the drugs and gave me more instructions about Mr. Thin and told me to ring her should I require any help. As I was the night runner, doing relief and there was a nurse off sick, I had no help at all.

At eleven, sister told me that there was a night emergency on the womens ward and she would have to help there. This left me with more feeling of panic than I have ever known since.

The whole of the night I tried, in an ineffectual manner to save the life of Mr. Thin. Keep the catheter in 'situ'; take his pulse every half hour, try to stop him falling out of bed, to interpret his low muttering delirium and feed him with ice when he repeatedly cried for water.

I struggled with the breakfast porridge, which had to be put on in a double saucepan and cooked for hours (this on the ward kitchen). Tried to cut bread and butter for the morning and do the minor dressings, which had to be done at least twice during the night. I hoped and prayed that Jimmy would not travel, he made one half hearted effort and gave it up as a bad job.

Mr. Large, the man on the Carol Dakin's treatment sat in his chair with his feet in the bath, looking very much as I imaged some of the Prince Regents in the Georgian days must have looked. He dozed through the night and grunted in the truly 'cardiac manner'.

Mr. Dyer snored long, loud and lingeringly, night sister hurriedly came and went, giving me advice and went back to the other cases in the womens ward and to see the sick baby on the children's ward and to try and give comfort to the parents of the same baby (this ended happily).

When eventually the morning came and the cheerful life of the day began for most of them, Mr. Thin died. His relatives who had been in the hospital all night were there. We were taught to always treat them with kindness and consideration and to make tea and toast for them, should they require it. All this was done by the J.P.

The patient died just before I went off duty. We were taught to say a prayer for the dead and always to find some flowers and put one or two into their folded hands. I have never feared death as it always appeared to me to be part of living. Most people who have departed, grow young again and all the lines seem to fade from their faces and they look as though they have come to the end of a lane with an unexpected surprise there. They know; but we do not!

The crowning insult came from Mr. Dyer who said that he had not had a wink of sleep during the night.

I staggered off duty, looked in the mirror, my hair was white? No! it was only the wintry sunlight. It was still brown, wavy and had its copper sheen. Perhaps I would risk it and keep a date with Sam Chandler. It was not yet my night off but I felt that I had had sufficient of hospital life to last me for a long time.

Having decided upon this course of action, tired as I was, I rang him up and told him that I would meet him later in the morning and we would go out for a meal and I would spend the rest of the day with him. I enjoyed this excursion, much better than I would have done normally, as I knew that it was against all rules for any Pro. to be out after mid-day without permission. One thing I had not taken into account, was that the night nurses' home had a very high fence, made in the Victorian style. This had a gate which was locked after twelve thirty.

I did not know that I had been observed by a not too charitable member of the committee who lived over the other side of the road. She (never had been young I suppose) informed the Matron, that one of HER nurses had been seen climbing inelegantly over the gate.

Matron was justifiably annoyed that I had taken THAT way of coming in. For this escapade I had my next night off stopped and as we only had one a month, my next was not due till December. I had my next one late in January.

Disaster overtook me again. I had arranged to meet Sam at six in the evening and to stay at his home for that night. I asked the maid to call me at five p.m. to give me time to bath and change into mufi. We had arranged to go to a second house show in London.

I never knew what really did happen but I woke up, as I thought, in the evening, I looked at my watch. It said eight o'clock. I went to the window and to my utter amazement I saw the wintery sunlight filtering through the bare trees.

Having gone to bed at about nine thirty in the morning, I had been so tired that I had slept from then till eight the next morning. I am not given to wasting time regretting the past, but I always have felt that I had missed something. Beside which, it was very difficult to explain, that it was possible for one so young to be so utterly exhausted.

Once at Christmas time, I was determined to go out at midday and spend the rest of the day with Sam. Having a streak of obstinacy in me, I proceeded in a bold manner, (not over the gate) to the front door, when to my horror, I saw Flossie Flannel Feet coming in the opposite direction. It was just a matter of which one could move the faster. Necessity, made me the winner. I reached the door and was opening it in a nonchalant manner, when a voice said, "where are you going, nurse?" Turning to her I said "Xmas shopping sister" (this was partly true). She appeared so mad that she forgot to send me back to the home. Or DID she forget? I often wonder!

After the episode of my long rest, came the hospital ball. We poor night nurses were allowed to stay until eleven o'clock and then we had to return to the wards.

I had never been to a dance in my life, as dancing was a hobby that my parents frowned at, in the supposition that all such pastimes were the inspiration of the devil.

This did not deter me from enjoying myself and thanks to the kindness of the pretty Irish staff nurse and Sister Evans, I really did.

I had been going to sport an evening dress and accessories, but had no need.

One morning three weeks before the dance, I was handed a parcel. In great mystification I opened it and there was a length of material, in a heavenly shade of pink and with it, a necklace of pink pearls. Enclosed was a card,saying that it was sent hoping I would be able to have it made up before the ball. This I did.

I was delighted and dumfounded at the same time. Unfortunately we were then not allowed to take our own partners but had to be content to be patronised by the honourary medical staff and the big noises of the committee (which was all important). Woe betide the Matron who was foolish enough not to keep on the right side of those august beings.

It was funny to see a tall, bald headed, middle-aged man trying to unbend to a small timid Pro. who perhaps like me, as yet had never been to a dance.

We did not like being talked down to, by what was to us in those early years, an OLD MAN! (Looked at with the cruel eyes of the youth.)

Katie was lucky as Percy, (who belonged to the elite) was there with his uncle. As they both danced together with great enjoyment and Irish abandon, there were many curious and envious glances directed to them. Katie with her shining wavy brown hair, shining dark eyes and her flame coloured dress, (sent by father who must have been paid in material instead of fowls). However she was a lovely sight and Percy, was in one of his best moods and out to enjoy himself.

I went back to the duty of runner and it was my job to go and relieve on the children's ward, while the staff nurse had her few hours at the dance. It was then the end of the old year 1930 and in a few minutes it would be 1931.

I could hardly believe it but I had been at the W.G. only seven months. To me it seemed a life time.

I have had many such lifetimes to pass since then. One morning in February, I was still on night duty and felt that I had just had enough of night duty, lectures, nappies and toilets of all kinds. Everything connected with sick people had a deep repulsion to me. Not even Katie could cheer me up. Of Sam, I had seen only little and Mr. and Mrs. Chandler were a myth and I secretly began to agree with all the pessimists who said that nursing was an awful life for a young girl. I hated the look of the patients, every one of them appeared to me to be more comfortable and felt a lot better than I.

This state of affairs, happily for me, came at last to an end. This particular morning was lecture day. This meant that after the morning meal and before I could fall into bed, we had a lecture from Sister Marshal. I plucked up my courage and went to her, with the request to be allowed to be excused, as I had a bad headache and sore throat. She was in a pernicity mood and said, "I shall have to take your temperature". She flounced off to fetch the thermometer and came back, stuck it under my tounge, in such a manner as though to say, 'that will catch you out'. But it was her turn to be alarmed, when she gazed at it, her face registered acute concern.

"Stay there until I fetch Matron!" This is the last I remember for a while. My next memory is of being in bed in the sick room and a swab being taken of my throat.

I heard after that my temperature had been one hundred and four and the elderly physician who came to me had diagnosed diphtheria. This was confirmed when the result of the swab arrived. I was packed off to the isolation hospital. It was the only time in my life, that I thought I would die and I did not mind in the least, I felt I should make my will and my possessions go to my mother.

I did not have to go to this trouble, as a few days after I had been injected with anti-diphtheria serum I started to take note that I was still in the land of the living and even felt HUNGRY.

In nine weeks I was back on duty again. While I was off sick, our Matron achieved her ambition, that each nurse should have half a day off a week and two evenings a week and a day off a month. Most important of all the off duty had to be made out by the ward sister and displayed for the nurses' benefit. This had to be done a month in advance.

This was great, no more being told the same morning at ten o'clock.

We were in Paradise!

CHAPTER 7
"A Serious Illness"

I found it to be a totally new experience to be the patient and not the nurse.

I learned what it was to lie in bed with no pillow. In this position I was expected to lie in a docile manner and accept the administrations of a nurse who had as little experience as I.

In the first week I suffered all the indignities which, for the first time made me realise what some of my own unfortunate patients had to thank me for.

There were those who made our beds, coolly, efficiently and impartially, without imagination, just as though they were packing sardines in a tin. They did the right thing at the right time, correctly and as they had been taught.

These had never had the experience of trying to balance themselves on a bedpan, which by the way, were of the old fashioned type, known as the "frying pan". My unfortunate neighbour in the next bed had the embarrassing experience of tipping it. She (a nurse from the hospital where Percy was officiating) had been allowed to do without a draw macintosh, until now, but as a result of this incident, we both had to lie on this uncomfortable piece of hospital bed-ware.

The most disappointing thing that can happen, is to imagine that you are going to enjoy a cup of tea. This is impossible as the article which is presented to you, is like a teapot and somehow it always tasted of carbolic.

The other indignity is to be wakened up at four in the morning and to be given (by a very new and apologetic nurse) an enema, this felt very cold, to add insult to injury. I grew cunning and so managed to do without and always had a dose of epsom salts on my breakfast tray which was always attractively laid. So this also, was a snare and a delusion, but infinitely better than the former type of treatment.

After a week I was allowed a pillow and life looked a little more rosy.

As I began to recover (despite my treatment) from the effects of this most unpleasant disease, I began to see the patients point of view. I had my likes and dislikes. Nurse Proud was one nurse who I actively could not bear to have near me. You, who have never been left to the tender mercies of nurses of diverse characters, cannot be expected to understand. She had the habit of taking our pulse with the extreme tips of her fingers and it was as though a cold cod had suddenly sprouted hands, MOST DISCONCERTING. Her manner to poor Molly and me gave the impression that we were in the advanced stages of leprosy.

Later on it was explained to me that we (the two nurses) were suffering for the sins of others. Just before we were admitted, there were discharged from this ward, two nurses from another hospital. These had been treated as private patients and had the same kindness shown to them, as we did. After leaving, they had complained to their own authorities that they had not been treated (THEY thought), in a manner, which was their due.

Nurse Proud had not recovered from this. I began to realise what nursing was. The hospital admitted more children than adults. I lay and watched, with what care they treated the poor little scraps who, perhaps had not been diagnosed early enough as diphtheria for the serum to take active and quick effect. Often the parents had reluctance to send for the doctor because they had not the where-withal to pay him with. (Most did not expect payment).

Late or early, as soon as they were admitted they were given massive doses of anti-diptheric serum. This did not always save the little life. Many times I awoke in the night to hear a muffled activity in the usually minute theatre at the end of the ward.

Usually it was the case of a child brought in nearly asphyxiated, with the membranes of it's throat inflamed, swollen and blocked up with it's own mucous.

A tracheotomy was performed and the patient had a fifty-fifty (much less!) chance of recovery, if it's heart could stand the pace.

I had had the disease when I was eight years old and it was considered very rare to catch it twice. As this was true of me I came to the conclusion that I had contracted it through being very run down and a few days before I was admitted, one of the little boys on the children's ward at the W.G. had developed the symptoms of it and had been rushed off to the isolation hospital.

Our old physician, who had attended me at first came strolling down the ward, with a message from our Matron. What did I want. All I could seem to think of was blackcurrant jam. Most ordinary, but duly delivered. We had no visitors but I had the satisfaction of knowing that Sam called at the enquiries with letters and fruit and above all, BOOKS, without which life would have been barren as a desert.

I was allowed to get out of bed in the fourth week. It was the worst thing that ever happened to me. I could not stand, much less walk. My legs were like chewed pieces of string. Poor Molly was as bad. We made a heroic sight as we pushed a chair in front of us, to help. I was just thinking that I should be allowed to go home, when I was stricken with a severe attack of tonsillitis. This condition was to haunt me at regular intervals all through my training.

Only after I was S.R.N. and a staff nurse at the mature age of twenty four, I had these offending parts of me removed.

Molly and I were discharged on the same day, she to her hospital and I to mine.

We bathed in carbolic and washed our hair in Durbac soap. We then dressed in our clothes, which had been sent. After this the taxi arrived and my favourite, Swiss staff nurse waved us off.

Having reached my own hospital, I was paid all the salary that was owing to me. Then the same taxi took me straight to the station. I could not stay the night at the W.G. in case of infection I was told. It was very ironic that the public could be so exposed. As they could not know the danger they MIGHT have been in, this did not matter.

I caught the next train to a terminus in London and then on to my own home, two hundred miles away. When finally I arrived home, I was nearly in a state of collapse and as my family did not expect me until the next day, it was a surprise to them in more ways than one.

After three weeks convalescence, I returned to the William Garrett. I felt as though I had lived through a strange era. However I was still only nineteen and as I began to feel stronger, life assumed a more normal aspect.

Katie Susan was delighted to have me back again and I was dying to hear the latest news of her romance.

Even Nurse Rochester seemed glad to see me. Years have passed but I can still see the picture of the lovely mauve tulips that she had sent me when I was in the isolation hospital. They were a complete surprise, as it was February and deep snow was outside in the world, (which seemed so far away). I have never forgotten those flowers or her.

CHAPTER 8

"A Visit To The Theatre"

When I looked at the duty list, I was surprised and delighted to see that I had been allotted to the theatre. I felt very jubilant about this move and the next day Matron came to me and said that I would not find it so hard, she thought it would give me time to recover from my illness.

I can look back to this period of my hospital life, as being pleasant and fairly uneventful. This in comparison to working on the wards.

While I was away, Katie had done a short spell on "nights" but was now on the children's ward and enjoying it. We were still sharing a room and when we were off duty she catechised me as to my store of knowledge. She would sit up in bed, a study book in her hand and spectacles on the end of her nose (these she had to wear to read with).

Although she never passed her State Prelim, owing to her fear of exams, which caused her to have stage fright, she was determined that I should pass and be a credit to the W.G. and our Matron. At that time we did not know what a scurvy trick fate was to bestow on Percy. As it happened it was just as well that she was not too ambitious, for as her life was bound up with his it proved, as you shall here later, to be in the hat.

As I was undressing, or combing my hair she would devour chocolates, supplied by Percy or Sam and shoot questions at me, these I had to answer whether I wished to or not. It had to be correct, if not, "you'll never pass if you go on like this" she would say. "Describe the respiratory system", was one of her favourite questions. Strange as it may seem, when eventually I went to take my Prelim. the first compulsory question was "describe in detail, the respiratory system and describe the portal circulation". This was another of her pet questions. Thanks to her, I found this to be child's play.

Fortunately the first day on the theatre was a Sunday and Sister Fairhurst took the opportunity of introducing me to sterilisers, both for instruments and dressing drums. These I was told, I had to learn to manipulate. The cupboards were full of shining instruments; these resembled carpenters tools and some Oh! horrors! reminded me of the butchers shop, the only difference was that they were much more refined and it was one of my duties to clean and polish them. Woe betide me if a speck of a foreign body was found.

There were hammers, mallets, saws, fret-saws of all sizes. There were curious instruments called retractors, ranging from tiny eye retractors to large ones to deal with such sizeable women as Mrs. Cherub on the women's ward.

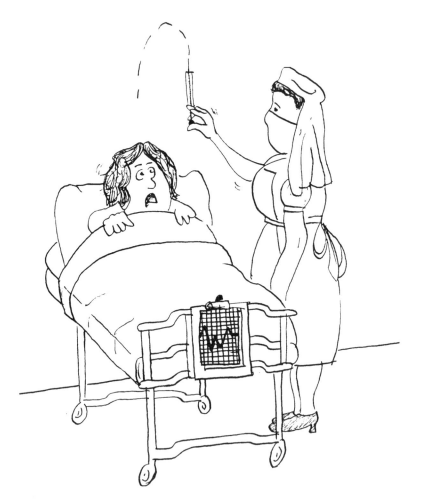

"This will make you better"

"Familiarity breeds contempt" and in due course of time, continual washing, boiling and cleaning of them bred this in me. I became on such terms with them, that I called them by their Christian names. On the Monday morning, staff nurse instructed me in the noble art of "squeegying" the theatre floor. Clad in a white overall, white gumboots and a turban on my head, she showed me how to fill a bucket of water and flavour it with Lysol. This I had to throw in a manner similar to a seaman swabbing the deck, as the floor sloped very slightly, the water found its own level, to the drain. There was, or seemed to be, an art in using the "squeegy". It was a peculiar mop which was rubber and until I was used to it, it had a habit of sticking to the wet floor and would not budge. I became very proficient with this creature, it made me understand what a lot of good is done by allowing small children to play with water and sand or mud. It gives a delightfully uninhibited feeling.

It seemed in my first year that however I tried I could never escape the inevitable laundry. Even in this envied position of "dirty nurse" (as we were known) I had all the sluicing of the theatre towels before they were sent to the laundry. These were in those days, all white. We did not have any call for green ones. Many theatres since, have adopted this more restful colour.

As I have mentioned before, we had no resident doctors, so apart from emergencies, which were treated by the doctor and surgeon of the month, each G.P. and surgeon had their own operating day.

We had no proper anaesthetic room so the patient was brought straight into the operating room, with only the pre-medication which was given on the ward.

I remember one patient who was brought in to have a repair of a simple hernia. He gave the anaesthetist a hot time, he roared with laughter and the more ether he was given, the more he laughed and laughed. Chaliapine singing and laughing in "The Song of The Flea" had no comparison to this weedy little Cockney. "If only Fred were 'ere', e would'nt 'alf larf'e, would'e, would'nt 'arf larf, 'e would, Ha! Ha! Ha!" At last he was quiet and his operation proceeded uneventfully.

We had two lady honoraries, who practiced locally as G.P's. One gave the anaesthetic, while the other operated, if necessary. Both of them were middle height and middle aged, their features undistinguished. They made up for it with their hats. As they wore severely tailored suits, these were all the more noticeable. One day, they arrived with a bunch of flowers on their heads, or one would have a thing shaped like a Chinese coolee's head gear. Sometimes it would be an inverted mushroom, which would detract from their short stocky figures and hide them completely.

It was always a speculation to guess which hat would appear, or what the latest creation would be like. Sometimes we would start operating in the morning and go on until late in the day. As this was often the case, I was lucky and had a lot of evenings free. On these days, I would be hurrying and scurrying about, from the time I came on duty until six o'clock, having rinsed all the soiled linen, ready for the laundry, washed, boiled and dried the instruments and put them away in the cupboards.

If a surgeon did not approve of a scalpel, he did not say so in any polite language but threw it into a tray with a loud crash. If an instrument did not suit, he simply threw it across the theatre, to be picked up and cleaned by the "dirty nurse".

I often was of the opinion that if the surgeon had had a difference of opinion with his better half before he came out, it was one way of letting off steam. It released his inhibitions and did no one any harm.

If there was a long operation and I had finished doing all the routine chores, sister would call to me and tell me to get as near as I could to see what was going on. As I am very short, I had to stand on a stool. The surgeon, if he realised I was near, would kindly try to explain what he was doing. Under my swaddling clothes, my mask and my cap, I would try to look intelligent, I did not find it very easy.

During those three months on the theatre, I saw many kinds of operations. These included appendicetomy's, hysterectomy and mastoidectomy. I saw one of our well known industrialists have a trepanning to his skull, to remove the pressure of a cerebral abscess situated under the bone. To my knowledge he is still alive and flourishing, making millions to die and leave to others.

One operation we used to do on a Tuesday afternoon was tonsillectomy and commonly know as T's and A's. This in the year of our Lord 1931, was not a pleasant affair. It was treated in a light hearted manner that is sometimes adopted by those who have never been the victims.

The parents of the unfortunate children were sent a card to say, "Would they give their child a dose of syrup of figs on the evening prior to their visit to the hospital". Added to this, they were told to give a light early breakfast of tea and toast at some ghastly hour of about six o'clock a.m. Then the child would according to their upbringing or nature be silently apprehensive or uninhibitively noisy. The tearful mother was then told to go and return at about 4 p.m. complete with blanket or chair to carry the child home.

They were taken to the out patient theatre, one at a time, given a light anaesthetic and the tonsils were guillotined and the adenoids removed. By the time this was done, the child was coming round from the anaesthetic and was roaring his or her head off.

As theatre nurse it was my duty to do the usual clearing up. Another Pro. was given the unenviable job of carrying the infant into a room which was optimistically called the recovery room. The only furniture in there were a dozen straw mattresses which the children lay upon. They were supplied with kidney dish and a bowl of swabs with which in theory the Pro. was supposed to wash the patients face. The children were all yelling themselves hoarse. Not I think because they were hurt so badly, but with bewilderment and fright. The whole room was permeated with the aroma of stale blood, chloroform and ether. As I write this, after the passing of all those years, I still remember the hot summer days of that year. Although now I am far from any theatre, faintly, like the passing of a dream, I fancy I can smell those odours.

At the appointed time, the mothers would arrive, with blanket, push chair, pram or car, according to their means and status. At the sight of their child, by now washed and as clean as the nurse could manage, but looking somewhat pale, the poor souls eyes would fill with tears and this sympathy would communicate itself to the child who would then set up another yell. Sister would give the mother what advice she could, tell her to give the patient ice-cream and cold fluids for a few days. She also warned her, that if there was any bleeding from the throat, to bring the child back at once, first if possible to let the G.P. know. It did not often happen, but at times a child would be brought in and would be taken in the middle of the night, to have the bleeding vessel tied.

This rather barbarous practice was to cease gradually, all hospitals began to have the children in the evening before and kept them in the children's ward for three days after, according to their needs and age.

The old method had nothing to recommend it and I have been glad to see its passing.

The sister was very kind to me and taught me much. Although I have worked in the operating theatre many times, in a more senior capacity, I never thought it was my favourite kind of nursing. This was because I liked being with people and administering to their personal needs.

It was just like handling inanimate objects, it is a good thing that all of us think differently.

But to return to my life at that time. I am reminded of the old saying "Satan finds some mischief for idle hands to do". One day during a slack period, the staff nurse was instructing me as to the uses of various drugs and happened in her discourse to mention that a very weak solution of Atropine was used as eye drops. From this, she just mentioned that actresses were in the habit of using it to make their eyes look large and luminous. (I never found out whether this be true).

However, I am almost ashamed to say, that one Sunday afternoon when I was on my own in that theatre and I had cleaned all the instruments, polished them and lay them on their shelves, gleaming and beautiful, I became bored. I then directed my attention to the eye cupboard. In it was a very small bottle of Atropine sulphused as eye drops. Without thinking about the consequences, I quickly soaked a swab with it and rubbed it on my eyelids.

I do not know anything as to the theatrical profession and how their eyes react to such treatment, but mine began, in a few seconds to grow misty and in a little while I was almost blind. Before I reached this stage, I looked in the mirror and my eyes, which are normally large and blue were no longer so. They had increased in dimension and to my horror the pupils were dilated to the size of the Iris. They were like two shining pebbles.

As I went to tea, I met staff nurse, who took one look at my glorious optics and said, "you have been touching the Atropine". Stoutly denying any such thing, I passed on hurriedly to the dining room, where I kept my eyes discreetly turned to the ground and tried to efface myself in a manner not usual to me.

Luckily it was my evening off and Katie and I were booked to go to a concert, the proceeds to go to help and support the hospital. We sat at the back and I was able to keep my eyes closed. She helped me back to the nurses home, I felt like one who had drunk too much of the wrong liquor, at the wrong time, wrong place and too often.

In a couple of days, my eyes were normal again and sufficient to say, I never dabbled in that kind of beauty treatment again.

I passed through the period of time which I spent in the theatre, in an uneventful manner. I know that it is contrary to the usual idea, but when eventually I was transferred to the children's ward, I was glad. I felt like a prisoner who had been released from solitary confinement.

CHAPTER 9

"In The Lift"

On the same day as I reported to the children's ward, Katie was transferred to the theatre, to take my place. I think she enjoyed it more than I. It meant that she came in contact with her future uncle-in-law, also Percy was in the habit of visiting the theatre to learn from the mistakes made by his respected relative.

The sister of the children's ward, was a Canadian woman. She was a large bovine looking person, middle aged and inclined to sag in most awkward parts of her anatomy. Her lank hair was turning grey, her skin was sallow and she made no attempt at adornment. Her one claim to beauty was a pair of very dark brown eyes, which had a hint of sadness in them.

When first I went there, I seemed to spend my life trying to evade her. In this, I had little success. She was a martinet, only the best was good enough for her. Nothing seemed to escape her eye, that is, no mistake. To me at the time, she appeared to be a very irritable woman and bad tempered.

In the ward were twenty four beds and cots. The children admitted were in age from a few days old to fourteen years. The older ones were in a little extension at the end of the long ward. Unfortunately for the sister of this ward, she had a bedroom on the other side of the wall and if the babies cried at night, she had no sleep either. This could have contributed to her irritability. I never found out why this arrangement had been made but I can only think that at the time when the place was first built, the one in charge, had to be on call, by night as well as day. We admitted children with all manner of complaints, both surgical and medical were mixed happily together. The diseases ranged from gastro enteritis, (which even today still takes its toll of young babies and children), pneumonia and meningitis, which in those days was almost always fatal. The introduction of M. & B. was still to be made a few years later. Anyone who has heard the cry of a child suffering from this complaint will never forget and no nurse, can listen unmoved to the meningeal scream of all the contractions of the muscles which make the heels meet the head, they are heart rendering to see and to hear. To those backroom boys who persevered with their experiments for the good of humanity and succeeded at the 693rd one lies the removal and relief of this dreaded scourge.

There were those who had the common and garden bronchitis and spent their days of illness in the traditional steam tent, this being made by covering a clothes horse with blankets and admitting the spout of a special kettle made for this purpose. As there was no other treatment, this meant a long stay in the hospital and in time, the child would become part of the ward and if old enough, would know more than the new Pro. who would be always told by the said child which and what to do.

Many were the children admitted with appendicitis, mastoiditis, compound fractured femurs and other bones. All these were operated on and were treated with efficiency and kindness. I never heard an unkind word to the children from Sister Bird.

Staff nurse, there at that time, was a girl of twenty four, trained at one of the hospitals in a university town. She had a calm and pleasant personality. She took all in her stride and was a good teacher. She was well mannered and was quick to praise as to blame. Her reason for coming to our W.G. was that there was very good experience to be had, as we were not a teaching school for the doctors. Almost all of our staff nurses came and stayed one or two years and then applied for sisters posts at other places.

After Nurse Rochester, I think that Nurse Blair was one of the best. It was she who tried, I am afraid unsuccessfully to train me out of my worst habit, that of forgetting small things.

Once she told me, more in sorrow than in anger, that I did a lot of big things well, but forgot the details.

There was little Tommy Atkins who came in with a fractured femur. He was eight years old and never had a square meal in his life. He had all the perkiness of the born Cockney and all the courage that often goes with the life of independence in which the children of slumland are reared. When we took him in a lovely dinner, which we were convinced would make his eyes sparkle, we were greeted with loud yells of "take it away, I want fish and chips," or loud cries for bread and jam and like Rachel of old, "he could not be comforted"! As a contrast to this boy, was a girl of thirteen, Josephine by name. She was an orphan from one of the schools, supported by the Freemasons. Her operation for appendicectomy, worried her not in the least. She called loudly (and in no uncertain terms) for her drawing block and pencils, she then proceeded to question all the Pro's as to their boy friends, or any other hobby they may have indulged in. She then drew (in cartoon manner) the story of that particular nurse. Many years later, I heard of her, she had become a fairly well known artist.

It was a wonderful sight to see the babies, who had been admitted to the ward, suffering from the debilitating diseases, due to infection from insanitary conditions and bad or wrong feeding, gradually become fatter and looking less like small monkeys. The pity of it was, that a great many belonged to poor homes and so often returned to us, in a similar plight.

One evening, I was taking temperatures and I came to "Little Audry". (No! not the one of the laughs) but a baby of a few weeks old. She had been admitted with Marasmus (a condition causing wasting) and was now on the road to recovery. This made me all the more surprised as I looked at the thermometer, as it registered 109°.

I checked it, re-checked it and sent for the sister, who did likewise. She in turn sent for the doctor, who repeated the performance and thumped, prodded and listened, all to no avail! Little Audry totally indifferent, gurgled away quite happily and refused to give up her secret.

Her temperature subsided as quickly as it appeared. She lived and no explanation has ever been given of this phenomenon.

I grew to love and understand the children, for whom such women as Sister Bird, gave up most of their lives. It is thanks to her that many of us are alive and well today.

My junior (by very little) was Jane Brodie. She was a hard working and conscientious worker. She had the Yorkshire characteristic. In everything, she was thorough. Never did she skip anything that could be skipped. She had to "bottom it". As I have mentioned before, this was to carry her to great heights in the nursing world, but this was many years later.

Even Jane, despite her severe upbringing, had a mischievous streak in her. Neither she nor I, had sprouted wings and we were delighted to find a service lift. This we utilised to our own amusement. It was used to bring meals, letters and parcels.

It was worked by pulleys of rope and when sister and staff nurse were at dinner we hit upon the idea of a little diversion. We gave each other rides up and down in it. Childish? Well! One day in particular, Nurse Brodie was curled up in the lift and I was pulling her up when suddenly there was Matron's head, just below the level of the floor of the little lift. Hastily I went to meet her and I listened to her with apparent unconcern. Hoping that my face was full of innocence and attention.

"There was a baby being admitted in a few minutes, to be prepared for theatre. He had swallowed the badge from the apron of his nanny. "Will you see that the cot and everything is ready by which time the sister will be back from dinner". "Yes Matron" and with a sigh of relief I watched her go back down the stairs. Jane thankfully scrambled out of the lift. We were a little more careful next time. The baby proved to be a lovely boy of six months old. It appeared to be in looks, much more that its real age and despite the anxiety of it's parents and the poor nanny, (who had hard work to retain her tears) he chuckled away in an unconcerned manner.

He was taken to the theatre and as the badge was undone, they opened his little tummy and there it was. He made an uneventful recovery and went home with a much chastened nanny. But it was a thing that could happen to anyone. We all felt very sorry for her.

It was while I was on night duty that I experienced my first terrifying attack of night nurses paralysis. It is called this, for want, I suspect of any better name.

I had been sent to the childrens ward to special a boy named Derrick. He was eight years old. He had had whopping cough while at home and then he developed broncho-pneumonia, which had responded well to our attentions and then to crown it all, he had developed Measles, so had put the whole ward in quarantine. As the result of this, the ward was closed to admissions. Fortunately no other child caught the disease, so they returned to the bosom of their respective families. This left Derrick, he was not well enough to return, so while the ward was being fumigated, he was put in a side ward. This meant that a nurse had to sit with him, all night. As he slept, well, the poor nurse had to sew bandages and gamgee jackets.

By one o'clock, I had finished all that the day sister had left for me and was vainly trying to take in the advice of one of our most famous writers of nursing techniques "Doctors May" she wrote, "But NURSES NEVER!" Never what? I thought in a tired manner. Never what, never what! What was it that Doctors could do that I could not. At last I grasped it. They could make mistakes. They could diagnose. They had to! On their heads was the results there of. Well or ill. Good or bad. Dead or alive. Ours not to reason why, ours to do or die!

I soon tired of this and took out a volume of Pickwick Papers and lost myself to the trials of Mr. Winkle as he rode to Dingle Dell. The fire was comforting and the chair too comforting.

Any idea of sleep, would have horrified me. Sister was due in a few minutes on her 2 o'clock round.

Suddenly, there was a roaring, as of a cataract of water, I sat there petrified, physically and mentally. My eyes were wide open, I could see but not move. How long I sat in this state I cannot say, but suddenly night sister appeared. "Nurse! you are asleep".

With this the spell was broken. I vigorously denied this accusation, but to no avail!

In the morning, I spoke to Nurse Blair and she then told me its name and said that many nurses were subject to it.

During the course of my career, I have had several attacks of this most unpleasant experience. But the initial one was the most frightening of them all.

I have since found, that printers and even seaman, e.g. Navigating Officers and anyone who is alone for a long time at night also suffer from this and I do not think there is any reasonable explanation.

My time on this ward was coming to an end and I was really sorry. I had grown used to Sister Bird and did not take so much notice of her moods and irritations. I felt that there was some underlying worry and sorrow, of which I knew nothing. Years later, I heard the story of her knawing anxiety.

During the time that I was on her ward, she had had acute pain of which she did not complain. She had been to a surgeon, who after many and varied examinations had reluctantly come to the conclusion, that she was suffering from an inoperable cancer of the liver.

At the time we all knew her and had to bear the blunt of her irritations, the reason of which we knew nothing.

She died very soon after I had left the W.G. She was not in bed very long and her age was only 45 yrs.

At the end of a year and a half, we took our junior hosps exam and to my astonishment, I was first in practical work and was duly presented with some text books as a prize.

I can only assume that I was the recipient of these, because there was little competition.

I only had six more months at the W.G. and my Prelim. to take. If I passed, I should be leaving this friendly small hospital at the end of the year. However that part of my life to me, seemed centuries away. With our new found liberty, i.e. a half day a week and evenings we were able to take advantage of many plays and as Sam Chandler was on hand to escort me, I am afraid to say, I took him for granted. However, my smug self satisfaction was to receive a rude shock. One evening as we were riding back from the city, by the Metropolitan, in a dream, I heard him tell me that he was going abroad, to S. Africa and he had the offer of a well paid and interesting post in Rhodesia. Then without any warning, "would I marry him, before he went and go as his wife?

I suppose at the time I was so engrossed in my own affairs and selfishly had had no thought for him.

Bluntly, I told him, that I was going to finish my training. We had arguments over the course of a few weeks and in the end, he went to S. Africa. Many years later I was to meet him and he was accompanied by his wife. I felt no surprise, that she was round, plump and rosy and they seemed utterly suited to each other and as happy as the proverbing larks. I do not think that his parents, Mr. and Mrs. Chandler ever quite forgave me, as I think they felt that I had some influence in his going abroad. This I felt to be somewhat unfair.

CHAPTER 10
"The Examination"

There was a great joy in the family of the O'Briens. Percy had passed his finals and Katie had become engaged to him. All appeared to be well. He was appointed to be a house-surgeon to one of The Honourary Surgeons in the hospital in which he qualified. Ironically as it seemed later on, he was taking a course in opthalmics and this was the way of gaining experience.

Katie was full of glee but still held to the firm idea that she had always had and that was "No marriage" until she had passed her State Finals.

On the strength of these happy events, she decided that it was about time that I was taken out of myself, as I was still brooding over the instability of Sam, leaving me without an escort and his determination to go to S. Africa, minus me. I am afraid that it was my vanity hurt, much more than any deeper feelings.

Suddenly she decided that it was about time that she visited a cousin once removed. This august person turned out to be a Mother Superior of a convent, about six miles from us. This place was also an orphanage. I think that her mother had written a long time ago, reminding her of this relation. I think that Katie wished to show off her newly engaged status to one of her family.

As I had never been in a convent, my idea of such a place was very sketchy, to say the least. I had a vision of nuns whose garments frou frou'd, as with quick urgent feet, they went about their duties when working or praying.

On this our chosen day, it was bright and sunny and we climbed on the top of a bus and soon reached the convent. This was a very large prison like building and did not to me, seem to add to its attractive appearance by two iron gates. We rang a large and old fashioned bell and awaited the results with kindly interest.

I had been briefed on the way, to say nothing of her failures and then to my dismay, she informed me that she had written to her cousin, telling her that I was her most wonderful friend and that I was an expert in the gentle art of tapestry and embroidery. As I hate sewing in all its forms and disguises this was the worst thing she could have wished on me. As I knew nothing of the art, this made me very apprehensive. The door was opened by a rosy faced happy looking nun. She said that we were expected and showed us to a comfortable room with a good fire in the grate. The door quietly opened and in stepped one of the most lovely women I have ever seen. Tall and slender, her smile was a thing to remember. In age about forty five, strangely she reminded me of Katie.

We had a beautiful hour, only one in the course of a lifetime but never forgotten. She rang a bell and in was brought a tray with biscuits, wine and coffee, all these delicacies soon disappeared, for no matter what state of mind we were in or what the state of our heart, our stomach! NEVER seemed to suffer.

She only lightly dwelled on the subject of embroidery but wished to know when I was to take my State Prelim. Having made a note of it in her diary, "We will pray for you and God will help you".

In theory I am not religious but it gave me a feeling of comfort to know that all those nuns were praying for me.

All these years I have treasured this small incident in my heart and the results thereof were passing strange.

Having taken our leave, we wandered off in time for a meal at our favourite restaurant and thence on to the pictures and back to the hospital.

I never saw the Mother Superior again but I heard of her through Kate. During the Second War (which was at this time nearly seven years away) the convent was severely damaged but most of the children were safe, thanks to the actions of the nuns and the Mother Superior. She was badly injured and never regained consciousness, having died as she lived, thinking of others rather than herself!

During the two years that I lived and worked in the W.G., many incidents occurred, some of which stand out as bright and new as the day on which they occurred.

This one had its origin during the time I first was on the women's ward. Its sequel about eighteen months later.

I had been sent to the theatre and had been told to stay to the end, as this woman was to have the operation for nephrectomy (removal of a kidney).

Mr. Giles made the initial incision in the skin and gradually, having tied every blood vessel as he worked, began to explore the cavity, preparatory to removing the kidney. As he gently handled the tissues in an effort to find the extent of the damage, his face became more grave and more grave. Finally, instead of going on with it, he began to suture the cavity.

Then very quietly and sadly he said "there is no hope for this woman as the growth is malignant and she is most likely to be dead in six months! it is inoperable".

As this woman was only thirty years old and had not long been married, this saddened us. However I returned to the ward with her and as far as the operation was concerned, she made an uneventful recovery. Doctor Brown explained it to the husband and when her sutures were removed, she went home but for a strange coincidence, I should never have known the sequel.

Just before I left this, my first hospital, I happened to be on the theatre in a slightly more senior capacity.

Mr. Giles was again operating and Dr. Brown giving anaesthetic, as they were talking to each other, suddenly Mr. Giles said

"Oh! by the way, Brown, what happened to the woman with the inoperable growth, of kidney?" Dr. Brown looked surprised. "Did I not tell you the story of what DID happen?" "No! What did?"

Then I heard, what seemed like a miracle, at the time. The husband, after a lot of thought and worry, had decided to tell his wife the truth. It was as though, sharing his knowledge, gave them courage and determination NOT to accept this decree as final.

So they began the usual search for a second opinion and spent more money than they could afford. Having met with no other answer to their problem, they went to a faith healing sect.

Soon after she had attended these sessions, she began to feel better and her general health began to rapidly improve.

Dr. Brown had made arrangements for her to be X-rayed and to the surprise of all concerned, the mass of Neo-plasm had totally disappeared and at the time of which I speak she had just been delivered of a bouncing baby boy.

Mr. Giles did not say much, except that the growth could not have been malignant, or grudgingly, perhaps the days of miracles had not yet passed!

I make no comment. I leave my reader to form his or her own opinion.

I was on night duty on this same women's ward, when another incident happened, this being of the type which could only occur once in a lifetime. It has given me a laugh ever since, whenever I think of it.

Attached to this ward, were two private wards, the patients being my responsibility. In one, was an old man, who in his day had been a well known trapeze artist and to add to his other accomplishments, was a ventriloquist of no mean ability, as you shall hear.

He had come to the W.G. to have an operation for a strangulated hernia. He was now, nearly in the convalescent stage and was very testy.

The night of which I write started in a most uneventful manner. I had done the round of bedpans, drinks, treatments, backs and after having had the drugs checked by Sister Evans was in the kitchen, preparing the breakfast trolley ready for the morning. All was quiet! Suddenly! there was a terrific explosion. Before I could recover my wits, there was another and another and so on until there had been six in succession. I dashed into the corridor in time to meet one of the "up" patients who had come to investigate.

In the corridor there was a cupboard, which was the hiding place for brooms and mops and other cleaning utensils. To my horror I became aware that as a trap to the unwary, a crate of champagne bottles had been placed on the top. There was a radiator under (or near) so the whole place was very warm, consequently, the corks had popped of their own violation.

To make matters worse, they had been given to the old artist in the private ward. He had presumably given them to be put in a cool place.

In dismay, I gazed at the liquid as it ran down the side of the cupboard. I decided to leave the explanations to the day staff. By this time it was mid-night, so with the help of the patient, cleaned up the mess, I retired to the kitchen once more to partake of light refreshment known as the "midnight" meal. I had not finished this repast, when I heard from the street outside, what sounded to me like "yodelling" and as this was a pastime which was very fashionable at the time among the youth of the generation, I took no notice. This noise was going on such a long time, that it gradually dawned on me, that if it was the lads coming from the dance, that they were a long time on this call of "the mountains". A nurse must only run in the case of haemorrhage, fire or death. (too late I should think for the last), but I dashed, as an awful thought struck me, the sound could only be coming from the room of the old man. So it was! He was purple in the face, as I had forgotten to pin his bell push to the pillow. To crown it all, he wanted a bottle of his champagne to be opened, as he had permission from his doctor, to drink it whenever he wished.

First I asked him how he had made the sound, which should have come in through other ward windows, come into the kitchen window. Then he told me what I had forgotten that he was a ventriloquist. Then we got to the the core of the proceedings and I told him the awful truth.

He called the unknown offender, a fool in no uncertain terms and then recited to me a little saying.

"He that is a fool and knoweth that he is a fool, is a wise man but he that is a fool and knoweth not that he is a fool, is a damn fool."

What curious things the labyrinth of the brain retains or rejects.

It was after this spell of night duty that I was sent to the men's ward and Katie was sent to take my place.

Now, unwittingly I had always been a pioneer for the present generation of nurses and I contended that because certain rules had been laid down for professional behaviour, there was no reason that they should interfere with our leisure hours.

Rightly or wrongly I would not be early for breakfast. I often preferred to have ten minutes extra in bed. The night sister would if she was not too busy, stand just inside the door of the dining room and mark in the book L. or E. as necessary.

To try and reform such a hardened sinner as me, the Matron had made it a rule, that if a nurse was late for breakfast more than once, she was to forfeit her half day off. So one week when I had been late twice, Katie crept down to the office when she knew that night sister was on one of the wards, she skillfully altered the L. into an E. and I was saved.

The reason given for this rule was that a nurse needed to be perfectly fit to carry on with her chosen profession and needed the time to eat meals in comfort and give them time to digest. To give Matron her due, I never heard of this treat actually being carried out, whether from lack of candidates or other reasons, I never knew.

At Christmas that year, I had been presented with a lovely black cat, he was taken from the tree, resplendent with a scarlet bow and presented to me by Father Christmas, who in a voice with a Scottish accent, said it was a good luck gift, in hope I would pass the Prelim. The voice was very reminiscent of "Old Whisky". This satanic animal was to remain with me, only till after I had sat the exam and then he mysteriously disappeared, never to return. As I am not over partial to cats, even stuffed ones I was secretly glad.

The dreaded day at last came, it dawned fine and sunny and I took it as a good omen. Three of us set forth to one of the London Polytechnical schools and thanks to Katie Susan I found the written work very easy. I saw Mary Ellen writing away with a fairest satisfied expression on her face but there was Katie, with a stunned expression, looking bleakly at her paper. The first question was "describe the function of the liver and the Portal Circulation and the next was to describe the respiratory system". These presented no difficulties! I finished my papers in good time and had a little time to look round the hall. It reminded me of an exam day at school. All the desks were neatly supplied with pen, ink and blotting paper. On the platform the leading lights sat in state watching for any cheating and for any requests for more foolscap. There was only one male nurse taking his exam with us. He looked like a "little petunia in an onion patch."

After it was all over and the time signal had been given, we all trooped out, feeling elated or depressed as our natures ordained. If we had been men, we should all have descended the first pub but as most of us had never been inside one, we went to our favourite poor mans restaurant, Lyons, and devoured steak and chips. As I have said before, we under all circumstances, were hungry, Katie was very depressed and would not be comforted. She said that although she knew all the answers, she could NOT express them properly on paper.

Also she seemed unaccountably uneasy, about Percy. I could not think why she was worried, after all, it was not the first time that he had gone for a few days with his uncle to a friend in Lincolnshire. It was one of his chief delights to go "shooting". Katie always said, that when she and he were married, that they need never go hungry, as he was such a good shot and even though they were only rabbits or hares, they were grist to the mill.

Nothing I said could lift the gloom and yet as I knew that Katie was possessed of "the sight", her depression began to affect me. Arriving back at the hospital, we were greeted by the usual spate of fatuous questions.

Mary Ellen and I met Sister Marshal as we retired to the nurses home and she seemed satisfied with the answers that we had given. Katie had retired very quickly as she was in no temper to be telling Sister of her failings.

Very soon we had to take the oral exam but before this took place, Katie's life was altered in the time it takes me to tell of it. A telegram from Mr. Giles to her briefly stated that Percy had had an accident and was in the local hospital, near to the house at which they had been staying. This was followed by a letter which said that he had had an accident whilst out shooting. With the party was a man, whose name should have been Mr. Winkle, as he could hit any target but the birds concerned. This time, with serious results, which bad as they were, could have been worse. His right eye had been injured and he eventually had to be told that he had lost the sight from this one. This to him was a blow from which, at the time, we thought he would never be able to recover.

Katie as soon as possible went to see him and she said that it went to her heart to see him in such a condition.

To Percy, it was death to his ambition, to be a specialist in opthalmics. At the time his father-in-law to be was in need of an assistant in his widespread practice. He was beginning to feel the march of time. Later on, when Percy had returned to Ireland, he was persuaded to enter General Practice with him, with the view to becoming a partner later.

Katie at last, was persuaded by Percy, that his need was greater than any hospital and if she would marry him soon, she would be a greater heroine than ever she would be, as a State Registered Nurse.

So just before Mary Ellen and I left for our new hospital Katie and Percy were married and after a short honeymoon they took up the threads of their shattered ambitions and in time wove them into a pattern of a different life. As there was soon a small Percy and a small Katie and a practice to be attended to night and day, they had not time to be living in regrets but I lost one of my greatest friends, as circumstances made it, that I have seen little of her owing to the ocean that lay between us. I still have a photograph of the two of us, as we were in the second year of our training. It seems to me as though it was only yesterday. I can hear her in my dreams, reciting her favourite song of the Emerald Isle, taken from the Shawl of Galway Bay.

't was short the night we parted,
Too quickly came the day,
When sad and broken hearted,
You went from me away.

To return to more mundane affairs, Mary Ellen and I set forth one morning for the Polytechnic to take the oral part of this State Prelim.

Mary Ellen had armed herself against any failure by carrying a text book. To boost my own morale, she bombarded me with questions, which I refused to answer. "Do be quiet" I cried at last in exasperation but she might have been deaf for all the notice she took.

"What is the difference between cows milk and humans milk" "I don't know and I don't care!".

"Cows milk has no lact albumin in it and human has!" No answer from me!

Eventually we reached our destination, we were ushered into a dark little room, reminiscent of Dickens days. I did not have long to wait, a little bell rang and I entered the holy of holies, which was if anything, a shade darker than the room in which we waited. Before I had time for my eyes to pierce the gloom, a voice said "Good afternoon Nurse, what is the difference between cows milk and human milk?" "Very quickly and brightly, I replied, "Cows milk has no lact albumin and human milk has."

The matron at the desk looked at me in an astounded manner as I must have looked surprised at such a question. I cannot remember much of the exam, as this coincidence had left me a little stupefied. I could not resist telling Mary Ellen and she gave me a self satisfied smirk.

Soon after this episode and when we had heard the result and our success, I went on my annual three weeks holiday. This I spent with my brothers, one of whom had passed his matriculation and was going as a cadet in the Merchant Navy. He was my favourite as we had spent so much time together, tramping the moors and exploring the dingles, the forests and ready for any adventure, real or imaginary that happened to come our way. The next time I saw him it was after I had left my training school and had the coveted S.R.N. after my name. I hardly recognised him in his uniform, he seemed to have changed to a man of competence and ability, in such a short time.

In the October following, two rather forlorn figures one tall and buxom, the other short and slim, set off to the station, waved off by all the staff (including Matron).

We had fulfiled their expectations and were the first Pro's to sit and pass the Prelim and to go on to the large Provincial Hospital in East Anglia. (This was the place where our Matron had been a sister). We were to meet other adventures but at the time, we felt like chickens who had been sent away from their mothers into the cold, cold world, of which we knew nothing!

CHAPTER 11

"A New Beginning"

Having waved good-bye to all the staff at the W.G. we set off for our new hospital. As far as I was concerned I did so with very mixed feelings. Mary Ellen was as usual talking. I think she did this so to cheer her flagging spirits. I remember very little of this journey, except to note what flat country we were passing through.

Gradually, Mary Ellen gave up her conversation and we passed the last hour in complete silence. If we could have seen our faces, respectively, I think we should not have felt any keen interest in them.

About ten miles from our destination we awoke and I noticed that there was a broad tidal river with small fishing boats on it. This scenery was new to me and I began to take a more active interest and to look forward to exploring some "fresh fields and pastures new."

It was not the best evening to see the first glimpse of this East Anglian town. The rain was coming down in torrents, so we spent some of our hard earned money to hire a taxi. In ten minutes we were deposited with our pathetically small amount of luggage on the imposing steps of the front porch.

We paid the driver and quickly looked around and what we saw impressed us, even in the driving rain.

It was a large building with the afore mentioned porch. This appeared to be built of white stone and had four massive pillars. The hospital was on top of a hill and had a sweeping drive with flower beds to each side. We were later to find these were a lovely sight, with varying colours in different seasons but at the time we were not concerned with the flora and fauna of the scenery.

Having climbed the steps, walking under this massive piece of Georgian architecture, we timidly negotiated the outer and inner door and hesitatingly approached a small cage-like edifice with the legend *Enquiries* above it. The large and impressive looking man in this box was in an imposing green uniform complete with gold buttons and war medals plastered over his chest.

Having finished a conversation over the telephone, he then condescended to look down at us, yes even down on Mary Ellen who was tall. He reminded me of my friend King but the great difference lay in his dialect. I was used to the pert Cockney and Mary to the Welsh language and like all Welsh, she had learned to speak a very pure English. This dialect was like nothing I had ever heard before and the whole time I was there I had difficulty in translating the words. This led me into some difficulties later, as you shall hear. Having tried to look intelligent, Mary interpreted his questions. "I suppose you are the new nurses? I will send you to the home sister. This he did and in a few minutes another porter

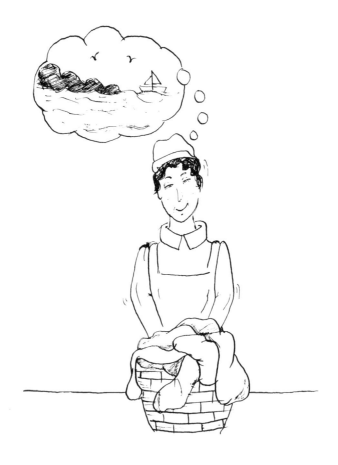

"Dreaming on the job"

appeared. His name he informed us was Jim. He took us through some underground passages; this way he said was used when it was raining. At last we emerged into the fresh rain soaked air, nearly to the door of the large nurses home. Later on I learned that it was known to all the medical staff and the local lads as the "Virgins Retreat". I have also learned in the later years that this title is not original but at the time I thought it was.

Jim rang the bell and deposited our luggage in the hall, grinned at us, winked at the maid who came and then departed. This being was dressed in black and wore her apron and lace cap, silk stockings and patent shoes in a manner which certain women wear mink coats. She looked at us with a very superior air, and if her nose had been long, she would have looked down on us. However, she sniffed and went to look for the home sister who proved to be a pleasant looking woman in a blue dress, white apron, army cap, blue belt and buckle of silver. Her eyes were bright blue, her manner mild and homely. Just the sister to care for a lot of over grown school girls, which many were.

Her name she said was Sister Charlesworth. She was in her middle thirties. We were taken to our room and introduced to a list of rules, which were made, as far as I could see, to be broken as fast as they were invented.

She apologised to us for having to put us in the old part of the nurses home. These rooms were dark and dingy and may have suited nuns in a convent. The mattress was about the most uncomfortable it had been my lot to sleep on. Even the buxom Mary Ellen was not comfortable. We had to put up with this place for three months and by the time Jane Brodie and Gwyneth arrived six months later, the new home was opened. This proved to be a luxury untold.

Sister Charlesworth then introduced us to two other Pro's and told them to take us over to supper and to report to Matron at 9 a.m. I was to go to the children's medical ward and Mary to the men's surgical ward. She gave us an encouraging smile and left us to the tender mercies of the two Pros.

These turned out to be two sisters. There names were Phoebe and Dorcas Wesley. Although they were not any relation to the real evangelist, they belonged to that Non-conformist Sect and were training as nurses in preparation for going as missionaries to darkest Africa. They were earnest and reliable, their faces round and well fed looking. Their figures, well, just plump. They had fresh shiny complexions and both wore spectacles. Their hair was long and mouse coloured and done in a style then known as earphones. This completed the picture of two lady missionaries as they were to become. I understand that there are different standards of beauty in different parts of the world, or even parts of the country.

I heard many years later that these two women did achieve what they set out to and eventually met and married two brothers, both missionaries, both as earnest as themselves and who both wore spectacles.

On this wet evening we knew nothing of these things. We were only too glad of their company to show us to the dining room.

We had our supper which consisted of stuffed onions, of which I was very fond, and rice pudding known as 365. The only day in which it was not served was Christmas Day.

Having reached the end of this exciting day we were glad to get into bed, even if they were hard as tramps palliasses.

I could not sleep at all for a few hours, there was strange noises, comings and goings, water being run, shouting and laughing. At last when all these sounds finished I fell into an uneasy sleep in which I was hearing Katie calling, "hurry up, hurry up, you will never get there, hurry up, hurry up." I awoke with a start to hear successive doors being banged, one after the other and the voice of the maid as she opened and shut the bedroom doors and shouted "half past six, hurry up."

We were unaccustomed to so many people about us. The dining room held twelve tables which seated five nurses on each side and one at the top. This was an unenviable position, as like the proverbial mother, had to do a lot of serving and this meant that her own meal was often cold. There was a long table well away from ours. This was the seat of the favoured few, i.e. the sisters and as they dined at different hours from us we never knew what delicacies they devoured. We knew that they did NOT have stuffed onions and 365.

The maids wore brown in the morning and had white mob caps. They were resplendent in black after 3 p.m., but I saw none to beat Christina.

I was taken to the children's ward by a Pro. who had been with me at breakfast. She was a pretty girl with a cheerful face. Her complexion was like a rose and her hair a light brown. This she used to wash and care for by rinsing it with the yolk of an egg. It was naturally curly. Her eyes were blue and kind looking. In all the times I was there I never worked on a ward with her but she became one of my best friends and we were to meet again in strange circumstances after twenty years had flown, when it seemed as though the years had never been. But this story belongs somewhere in another book and another end.

This morning I was only concerned with my introduction to this new life. Staff nurse was an Irish girl, trained at the Rotunda Hospital and was working for two years at St. Anthony's Hospital. She was very capable, but unfortunately for me, her two years coincided with the two that I had to complete to finish my training. It seems to me as though she dogged my footsteps, very often all of the time. She was a redhead and had a temper as hot as her hair looked. I called her Ginger and Ginger she has remained to me.

Sister proved to be a dear and loveable woman. No beauty and not young, but oh!, how those children adored her and how I have remembered her.

I remembered little of that morning as Mary Ellen and I had to report to the Matron's office. We waited in a room which we found to be the board room. This at the time conveyed little to us. We sat there looking at the portraits of the deceased governors of the hospital who all seemed to have been brewers. These were mixed up wit pictures of such men as Lister Simpson, Lord Monyhiam Pasteur, Marie Curie and of course Florence Nightingale.

Matron was a smart young looking woman of about forty. She hoped we would be happy and a credit to our former Matron and wished us well. We then returned to our respective wards. This sounds easy but was it? Every corridor promised to reach the children's or the men's ward, but we seemed not to get any nearer. At last we plucked up courage and asked an important looking being, dressed in a white coat. In a broad Scottish accent he told us that he would take us. He turned out to be the R.M.O. He was a heavy looking man in his early thirties. Sandy hair already turning grey and as far as I could see nothing to recommend him but his delightful Scottish accent. However, Mary Ellen thought otherwise.

When I came off duty that afternoon I had time to memorise all the rules for nurses.

We were to be called at 6 a.m. for breakfast at 6.20 a.m., on duty at 7 a.m. We were not allowed out after ten in the evening without a late pass from the Matron.

No nurse was allowed from the hospital in uniform. We had no official outdoor uniform so we had to change into mufti, even to go to the local tuck shop. This is one of the rules that to this day I agree with.

Every nurse had to make her bed each day. That meant strip and air it. Now, as all of us know, having had enough of making beds during the day, we just tidied them. This did not deceive home sister at all. I think she had a rota for each bed was periodically stripped by her, then we were forced to make them. These occasions were always when we were in a great hurry.

No nurse was allowed to leave the hospital grounds without a hat on. I never discovered the reason for this rule and most of us wore a pimple of a cap and when well away from the building took it off and put it in our pocket.

At first our new type of caps took us a long time to make up but I became adept at making these monstrosities for myself and others. They looked pretty on some, but on others I thought them to be hideous.

We felt lost in such a large place and it took us some time to get acclimatised to so many people and find our way around.

The virgins retreat housed about one hundred and sixty nurses and sisters. The hospital was not a teaching school for doctors and accepted about three hundred and sixty patients.

There were many honoraries and they in their turn had their own house surgeon and physician. The Resident Medical Officer I have already mentioned.

In the short time we had been there we had seen more men than we had seen at the whole time at the W.G.

The houseman wore short white coats and most of them had a stethoscope in their hands or coyly swinging from their pockets. I think this badge of their profession gave them courage, that I think some of them fresh from their own hospital lacked.

Of course, the great ones arrived in their cars, opulent or otherwise as their tastes, finances or their wives dictated.

Having been greeted at the front door by the porter, they sailed majestically to their own room. They then donned a long impressive white coat, that in the case of a short man, made him look shorter or a tall one look taller. Followed by their houseman they proceeded to their clinic, ward, theatre or any other place that awaited them.

In time they became people and characters to me, each with his or her separate ways, whims or fancies.

As there were no students, the nurses had a lot of treatment to do that would have normally been done by the students. I found that it was true, that this was a good kind of training and a very excellent experience. Many years later I have had cause to be pleased that I had taken these four years in a general hospital.

The children's ward to which I was sent took in about thirty children, from babies of a few days old to those of about ten or eleven. This ward only admitted medical cases, the surgical ward was underneath. On the balcony and the verandah were patients suffering from Osteomyelitis of various bones. There were also children who had T.B. joints. These were also nursed outside as soon as they had had their operation. Many of these children were encased in plaster. Some, if their spine was infected, had one from neck to toes. You might think that this impeded their movements. The treatment in those days was complete immobilisation, so I was very surprised when the new nurses home was opened and I had a room overlooking the outside of that wing, to see the children scrambling out of their cots or beds. There was little Johnny who was in plaster from head to toe. His face like a little angel when the nurses were there. As soon as their backs were turned, out he hopped. This he did by silently letting the cot side down. He would move swiftly to a bed at the other end of the ward and fetch a toy or a sweet and then return as unobtrusively as he had gone.

Those suffering from osteomolyitis were also encased in plaster with a window cut in it to allow the dressing to be done. Previously the child had been to the theatre and the affected bone scraped, dressed and plaster covered.

I found that when Mr. McPherson had first come to St. Anthony's he had been highly horrified to find that T.B. patients, even though surgical only, were all bundled together. He made it his mission while there to have it altered.

In the process he made himself highly unpopular with some of the older physicians who didn't see why things should be altered. However, altered they were and the T.B. children were sent to the local sanitorium. This gave us more beds for patients who would not occupy them for such a long time.

There was on our ward a little imp by the name of Freddie. He was only three and every time a porter came into the ward he would shout "Oh yeah and how? says the bull to the cow." All our efforts to train him in polite conversation were in vain. I am afraid the porters used to laugh and encourage him and one day, to our horror, he shouted his set piece, to what he took to be a porter, but it was a rather old maidish physician on whose shocked ears it fell. He looked at us with suspicion, as I think he thought we had trained this tender infant in his choice of verse.

The same Freddie also had a very sore nose which had to be treated by cleaning and applying a special ointment.

Staff Nurse Ginger was in the habit of taking the trolley and a Pro. and doing this simple piece of dressing. This was accompanied by shrieks of protest by Freddie, who did not submit tamely to this treatment. She did not mean to be unkind but was very impatient. The first time she took me with her she must have read my thoughts for she looked at me and said: "If you think you can do better, well, you can get on with it." This I did. There were NO YELLS.

My secret, I did not do it at all. Little Freddie dressed his own nose. I procured some orange sticks, cotton wool and a looking glass, gave the things to the little boy and told him what to do. In his fear of Ginger he did it well and soon his poor nose was healed. He was a lovely lad, with his large brown eyes and his fair hair. We were sorry to see him go home, the ward seemed empty.

I always felt that Sister Walters was like the nanny in the musical comedy who sang "Other people's babies and mother to none." In this I was right as she certainly never had any children of her own, but to my intense surprise, I heard later, that she was engaged to a sea captain. One of those who roamed the world in an unpretentious tramp steamer. Before I left he came home on leave and they were married very quietly and she went to sea with him.

When I saw him I was pleased. They were both bordering on

fifty years old, he being a widower and she never married I think that she had known him years ago and had cherished a secret love for him.

Their faces were shining with happiness and we all wished them well. The only pity was that she was too old to have a child of her own. She was better with children than a lot of women who say "I LOVE children" and pride themselves on their great usefullness, when in reality, they only love themselves.

The house physician on this ward was a mystery to us. Aged about thirty-five years he was a good many years older than the rest of the houseman, many of them were in their early twenties. He was six foot two in height, bald headed, pale, intellectual faced. His hands, more of the hands of a violinist than a doctor.

Rumour had it that he had a love affair. This was only supposition, we never found the truth. Sufficient to say, he never fell for the wiles of staff nurses or sisters. They tried their best but he went on his way with a remote detached air. This attitude repelled most advances and protected him like a suit of mail. With children he seemed a different person. His shyness he shed like a cocoon. The honorary of this ward was a short plain, quietly spoken, middle aged man. He looked more like a farmer than a specialist in the diseases of children.

I remember one night, Sister Walters had gone to supper telling me that a new baby was to be admitted and I was to prepare the cot for him. This I did and then started to do the usual bed pan round. Although it was the older children's bedtime, I put screens in front of the door and went into the corridor to the duty room which was just outside. I saw a very ordinary little man there. Before the poor man had time to speak I said: "You can't go into the ward, Sister is at dinner and you will have to wait until she returns." Then, being trained to be polite to all visitors, I offered him a chair. He meekly sat on it and I returned to the ward.

Twenty minutes later, Sister Walters appeared and in her wake, came the little man. He looked at me and a sly wink came into his eye. I had never seen him before but in acute embarrassment, I suddenly came to the conclusion that it was the great man himself. Following him came Doctor Simpson, I felt as though the best thing to happen to me was the earth to open and swallow me. It did no such thing.

Instead they disappeared behind screens and started to examine little Rachel Joseph, a jewish girl who had been admitted that morning. It was suspected that she had an abscess of the lung. Doctors Witherspoon and Simpson were anxious about this little child. Between them they decided that she had an acute infection of the lung, not an abscess. She eventually recovered after a long period of nursing care.

While they were seeing to this little child, the baby was

admitted. He appeared to be in the last stages of bronchial pneumonia and as antibiotics were at least three years away, and to us, undreamed of, we had no help for him but our own skilled nursing, oxygen, brandy and other stimulants.

The little soul was blue in the face and his breath was labouring in terrible harsh gasps. His nostrils pinched and dilating and contracting. It was time for us to hand over to the night staff. We were all to think that his little life should be lost when a little attention might have saved him, if given earlier. A steam tent had been fixed, the oxygen cylinder ready. The mother sitting in a state of suspended misery. She was trying to control herself but the tears were streaming down her face. The two doctors were making their way down the ward and we followed.

Next morning when we arrived in the ward, we as one looked to the corner of the ward expecting to see a vacant cot, when to our astonishment and pleasure, there was baby Billy, sitting up in his cot, gurgling and laughing, his colour no longer cydnosed and his breathing normal. His skin was a lovely rose pink and his blue eyes shone. It was a good day for us, even Ginger seemed to be a little more affable.

There is not a nurse who has watched a child suffer and not been able to give much help but is pleased to see what, at the time, is like a miracle.

I was also sent to the surgical ward on the floor beneath the medical. The sister was a young and good looking woman. Tall, fair and of a happy disposition. She light heartedly took charge. Strangely enough I can remember little of this ward. One character I can never eradicate from my mind was Gladys. Just Gladys. Eight years old, thin, pathetically skinny I should say. Her face, more that of an old woman than that of a child. Her features sharpened by hunger and that of a child who too early in life had seen the seamy side and had taken it all in her stride. She had had the responsibility of younger children and was a gallant child who had taken any number of knocks and no amount of bullying could subdue her spirit.

At last, nature had her way and Gladys was admitted to us with Empyema (pus in the pleural cavity) and she could not breath without excruciating pain. She was taken to the theatre and the pleural cavity was explored and then drained. This was done by inserting a long rubber tube into the cavity. This same tube had to be taken out and another inserted. This was done each day and the wound washed out. As the reader may imagine this was by no means pleasant for the little girl.

When I was on duty it was my job to do her dressing. Gladys came from a large family, as did I. Consequently we had a great deal in common. We conversed on many matters appertaining to the care of young children. When I had put the screens around her, I would start to tell her a fairy tale. This in a quiet voice, I related as I worked and the tube was removed without any difficulty. When I reached the stage to put it back I would try to put the maximum expression into my voice. "What DO you think happened THEN?" "Can you possibly imagine?"

"Have you put it back nurse, what did happen?" This all in one breath. By this time I too was holding my breath. It did not matter the offending piece of rubber was inserted and I finished my tale and Gladys was bandaged and comfortable as was possible.

She was with us a long time and eventually went home fatter and taller. After all these years I wonder if she is as perky now as she was as a child. I cannot see her in any other way.

CHAPTER 12
"Time For Lectures"

Our lectures were now on a much more advanced scale. We, i.e. the nurses in my class, had to take them from varying honoraries. We started with old Pop Witherspoon. He tried to teach us as much as he knew himself. This was impossible as he was a poor one to import his own knowledge. I do not know if we looked as bored as we felt. He read his lectures and droned on and on and on. We were forced to take down every word and then had the arduous task of copying it down again in our lecture books. In our company of fellow sufferers was one, who I will name Nurse McAdlebed. She had been a short-hand typist once upon a time. So now she took her notes in shorthand and unfortunately, for those who relied on her efforts, she made a great many mistakes owing to her misinterpretation of her hieroglyphics. To sister tutor's annoyance, we nearly all made the same mistakes.

I never felt too drawn into the medical side of nursing but I think his lectures put the finishing touches to my dislike.

Our sister tutor was an elderly woman, tall with a figure like a bundle of washing. Her hair was grey and straggly, her skin was high coloured. Her eyes were blue, kind and humerous. She, I found out later, suffered from asthma.

She had been trained long ago, at one of the best London hospitals and had a deep antipathy to our Hospital Examiner, who not only had written a book, which we were supposed to study from but had been trained at a rival London hospital. Consequently her lectures were punctuated by remarks such as "of course, in your hospital exam, you do it this way but we at St. Giles did it that way." During the course of her discourse I would hear some of the more irreverent nurses murmuring under their breath "We at St. Giles did it this way." Still, most of us had a liking for her, despite her sometimes caustic tongue.

In turn we took lectures from P. A. (otherwise Painless Paul). He was the Honorary Dental Surgeon NOT, repeat not, to be mistaken for a mere DENTIST. This was his most careful admonition to us, NEVER go to a dentist, ALWAYS a Dental Surgeon.

We had advice and knowledge poured into us by Johny Gaynor, the Gynaecologist.

Lectures from the V.D. specialist, Eye specialist, and the Ear Nose and Throat Surgeon and last but not least from Mr. Barber on General Surgery.

Of all the lecturers I loved him the best. I liked the way he insisted that we did not take notes, only headings. He said that he could not bear thousands of scratching pens. He was not popular with all the nurses, as he had a habit of pouncing on some unfortunate Pro. who was sitting half asleep at the back and asking: "You at the back, what do you know of the technique for such an operation?" The unfortunate nurse concerned would stammer and stutter: "I don't know Sir." "And why not pray? have I not just explained it."

He was about forty-five years old and married with four daughters, but that did not deter me. I absolutely hero worshipped him. I cared nothing for his caustic wit. I liked it.

The other Pros. when they found that I admired him would push me into the first row, so that he would be forced to pounce on me, which he did. "Go on Herbert, you sit there." To the end of his course of lectures I always did. I always answered him, even though I knew nothing of what he asked. I never admitted defeat.

Later, at a staff dance, much to some of the sisters disgust, he asked me to dance with him and not only once. I asked him why he always chose me to ask awkward questions, "I always seem to see your little face looking at me," he said. I was in heaven for a few days later.

His technique in operating delighted me. His speed, lightness of touch. His one cry when teaching was "handle the tissues as little as possible, never waste time by shocking the patient and by pulling off dressings by force, as you only undo the good you already have done and tear the healing flesh and retard the patient's progress.

This to some nurses may seem superficial advice but often since then, I have seen dressings ripped off quickly in the mistaken idea that it is better for the patient but this is not so. Those concerned can never have had an open wound and have never asked the opinion of the patient.

All the time I was at this hospital Mr. Barber took a great interest in me, much to the disgust of my seniors and would stop in the corridors and talk to me. He would repeatedly ask me my name, he never could remember it. This I thought not to be complimentary, until I persuaded myself that it could only be a method to hold a conversation, even though limited.

One Sunday morning, while I was still on the children's ward, Ginger, who was in charge that weekend, had unbent enough to be standing at 9 o'clock behind the kitchen door, eating ham sandwiches. I do not remember where the ham came from but there it was and there we were. I had a dirty apron on and was about to go to the nurses home and change it, as we always did at about this time when suddenly we heard alert footsteps hurrying down the corridor. An unheard thing at that time on a Sunday morning.

Ginger, her mouth like a double gumboil, and mine the same, gave me a push in the small of the back and I landed, barely on my two feet, right in the arms of my idol. If ever pride suffered a fall, then mine did.

He smiled down at me and asked if he might see little David

Price, who had been on the danger list and was that morning feeling slightly better. By this time, Ginger had swallowed her sandwich, had smoothed her apron, put on her cuffs, adjusted her belt to her slim waste and serenely accompanied him into the ward. I had retired with a scarlet face and full of mortification.

In my heart, I never forgave her but I was recompensed in full measure some months later.

I was on O.P.D. (Out Patients Department). It was Thursday afternoon and I had been told by sister to attend Mr. Walters in the Eye Clinic. Once again Ginger was my staff nurse. I had prepared the room for him and as he liked a cup of tea during the afternoon, I had placed the tray on a table and was well pleased with my efforts. Next minute the door opened and my satisfaction received a rude shock. There was Ginger, her face as red as her hair and her pale blue eyes blazing. "What have you put the tray over there for?" she ordered. I tried to tell her that I had not known where it should be and unfortunately, I had the merity to say that I did not suppose he would care one way or the other. Of course, this insolence from a mere second year Pro. made her more mad and she let rip at me. I was so astounded that I stood there and let her rave. She was standing with her back to the door and so did not hear it open. There was Mr. Walters and he stood and listened to her tirade. As she was facing me, even though I had felt so inclined, I could not warn her. He was one of her own countrymen and I felt he enjoyed it.

Suddenly she must have sensed something wrong and she turned. As Ginger always liked to stand well with any of them, this was too much. I retreated, leaving her to carry on with the clinic.

Never very popular with her, my popularity sank even lower. By some fluke, I never went to the eye ward but at the opthalmic lectures I felt interested as he told us that a great many of the patients were old and suffering from cataracts. They were set in their ways and the rules that applied to the surgical wards and in others, should not be drastically enforced in HIS ward. Many men and women were in the habit of having a glass of beer or some kind of spirit. He taught us to try and find out their tastes and in moderation, not to alter them. He was of the opinion that it made for a more speedy recovery. I have found this to be also true in many conditions of illness or accidents.

At last I was moved from my dungeon-like room and Mary Ellen and I moved, with not an iota of regret. My room was a palace compared with the one I had vacated. There was central heating and a wash basin in every room. The decorations were tasteful, and best of all, the architect had planned the home with plenty of bathrooms. It meant that we did not have to wait in a queue. There was a drying room, an ironing room, a kitchen, and a room which was especially for hairdressing, complete with a hair dryer. I mention this as I have not found all these things, which are now taken for granted, in every hospital. Some months later, when I went on night duty, I had to move to the top floor. This over-looked the park and was nice and peaceful all the week until Sunday at three o'clock when the local Salvation Army Band used to strike up. We appreciated this when we were on day duty, as they always "hotted up" the tunes and made a mournfully evangelistic hymn become a good jazz number. But when one had been awak-ened at that time it was fatal to try and sleep again. MOST ANNOYING.

The girl, who I have mentioned before, who had remained my lifelong friend, even though separated for twenty years, proved to have the name Naomi, which at the time I did not think of as strange but as mine is Ruth, I think this is more than coincidence. She had a fund of dry humour and we had a great many interests in common, these included walking in the country, swimming and anything to do with the open air. I think she, like me, must have suffered from slight claustrophobia.

One of the luxuries connected with St. Anthony's was a bathing hut at the nearest seaside place, about ten miles away. This we made full use of. On our day off, we took the first train to peb-ble beach, fetched the key from the caretaker and opened the door of the hut. It is strange to say that even though there were many nurses at our hospital, there seem to be few who took advantage of this concession.

The night before we put in a request to the housekeeping sister, who provided us with a picnic basket which contained plen-ty of everything to prevent us from starving. This included fruit, cheese, new bread, tomatoes, lettuce, butter, tea, biscuits and chocolate. It had always been agreed that Pros. earned too little money to afford to keep themselves from their salary, which at the time, for a second year, was two pounds a month. This princely sum was delivered to us on the first day of the month. At nine in the morning the telephone would ring and a voice from the secre-taries office would say: "will the nurses come to the boardroom for their pay. Half of us would troop down there and take our place outside the door. One by one we would enter. The hospital secretary would be there, sitting behind a desk, just like a deity. He gave us a patronising smile, as though he was parting with his own money. He would silently hand us a form to sign and then his min-ion would hand us a packet containing this princely sum. It was pointed out to any rebellious nurse who dared to express the opin-ion that we were badly paid and that it was sweat labour, that we had our training free and that we were supplied with uniform, sick pay and attention and board and lodging. Therefore the money that we were graciously handed was PIN money. This was true. I leave my reader to work this out for him or for herself. Naomi and

I, on the first day of the month, would spend part of our hard earned salary on a visit to the local restaurant where there was the luxury of a small orchestra. We thought that it was the height of dissipation and we ENJOYED it, as did a great many of our colleagues.

Every other month, Naomi would ask the sister of the ward to give her a half day off and a first half, till 2 p.m. and she would catch the train to the West Country where her fiance was a policeman. They had agreed to separate until they had both passed their exams. This they did and were married as soon as she had passed her State Final. On the alternate month, Eric would come up from the West Country and stay at a local pub and they would spend a long day together. It lingers in my mind the morning when Naomi, having washed her hair and rinsed it in a beaten egg to make it fluffy and shining, her prettiest suit on and her face shining with expectation and pleasure, sailed off down the drive to meet the train. In about half an hour she was back. Eric had not arrived. A little later a telegram arrived. He had been delayed by an accident, which had occurred a minute before he was off duty. He had felt it was his duty to make a statement and consequently had missed his train. We all felt shocked for her sake as such a thing had never happened before to her. Eric was a tall handsome figure and was of an ambitious nature. In due course of time he reached his goal, which was to a Superintendent. This after many years he achieved through hard work and interest. He is now a comfort to the virtuous and a terror to all wrong-doers.

Among the staff there were many nurses who I had never spoken to. We had our fair share of strange characters. There was a girl, who was short, square, pasty faced, her hair mouse coloured. I heard her speak only once. This she did in a guttural coarse voice. She had a name, which only a vodka drinker would understand. Rumour had it that she was a princess in exile, but as rumour is a lying jade, I was doubtful.

As at the time I had never heard the word and if I had would not have known the meaning thereof. It was lesbian. This might have applied to two nurses who had a crush on each other. They seemed to live in each others pockets. They would sit in the nurses lounge and would recline on the settee, holding each others hand. They were also known to send notes to each other when on night duty or were on diverse wards. One was round, plump and rosy, about thirty and the other was long, lean and hungry looking. A face with the unhealthy palour of those who suffer from too little fresh air and a morbid mind, etc.

We looked at them in disgust but at the same time, being only women after all, we found them a slight source of interest. I never found which was the man and which the woman, and when they passed their finals they went off together and we never heard of them again. By this time the hospital had received two other nurses from the W.G., one was Gwyneth Price and the other was Jane Brodie.

Mary Ellen was in the throes of a love affair with the R.M.O. As he was married, this was a very tricky state of affairs, especially as ALL the medical staff were RESERVED for sisters only. On the moral side of the state we felt we had to shield her, even though we disagreed with her. Of course, there were those who were only too willing to step into her shoes. As months later he went to the colonies with his wife, I think his love life had caught up with him and he felt that discretion was the better part of valour.

Mary Ellen revived enough to pass her exams and went to be a staff nurse in one of London's most fashionable clinics. As buxom blondes were wanted, she was the ideal one for this place. Two years later she married an ageing actor who had plenty of what it takes to make the world go round. Money and EXPERIENCE and the desire to appear younger.

CHAPTER 13

"Good Little girl"

The next ward to which I was sent was a large medical one. It comprised of two wards, one of which admitted male and the other female patients. Each had fifteen beds and a side ward for two. The kitchen was at the end of a corridor between the two. They were known as the Bailey and the Bannister Wards. The latter being the womens ward.

Sister of this domain was a rather unusual character. She was tall, slim, dark haired, blue eyes and her walk was stately. Her looks belied her real nature. She gave the mistaken impression that she was always serious and thoughtful. This was not always so.

She was very popular with the houseman and it was the duty of the junior Pro. to make sandwiches and coffee, ready for her favourite of the moment, to refresh himself with. When I arrived on the ward, the house physician was a tall auburn haired, pink faced youth, with a deceptively youthful face but, he was a remarkably good and interested doctor. They were both full of life, this doctor and sister but had the interests of all their patients at heart. Sister West was one of the most original teachers in the profession and she cared little for red tape and always used her own discretion. She taught us to think for ourselves. Later on she and Doctor Pearson became engaged and eventually married. He became one of the leading consultants in that part of the country.

We did not partake of this luxurious lunch, but were regaled with black treacle and Dutch cheese. This I at first took to be a very curious mixture but having tried the two together was agreeably surprised. Even if it were to have tasted of straw I think we would have eaten it as we seemed to always be in a state of semi-starvation. We were given good and plenty food, so I only put it down to hours of hard work and plenty of exercise.

I did not care for this type of work. It seemed depressingly free from any dramatic results, such as one encounters on the Surgical Wards.

I did not at the time realise that I was watching history in the making in the world of medicine.

I was taken to the kitchen where I was instructed in the gentle art of serving uninteresting diets, in an interesting way. By the year nineteen-thirty-three, deaths from diabetes were becoming rare, as the use of injections in and out of hospital was in England the rule instead of the exception.

When there were many diabetic patients, life for us seemed to be one eternal round of bedpans, urine testing, injections and diets. These seemed to consist of tomatoes, lettuce, eggs and meat.

We were taught the influence that colour exerts over jaded appetites. As the patients became tired of mounds of tomatoes etc., it is not surprising that Sister West's sandwiches were of the best in the hospital. The houseman enjoyed them to the full.

Have you ever tried to make raw liver look as though it was an aperitif? Well we did try our level best. The new era of those suffering from Pernicious Anaermia was dawning, but what did we know of this. It meant just liver. LIVER in cocktails, liver in sandwiches, liver in salads, liver paste, all raw liver. I never found a patient to be deceived with these disguises. But even they were not to realise that just round the corner was death to this treatment. It came in the form of an injection, named Anahaemin. This was given into the muscle and in decreasing doses till the patent was stabilized, and was the death knell of LIVER.

We were made to poultice the pneumonia patient with a substance call Antiphilogistine, now known as Kaolin. We sponged them every four hours, changed the inevitable gamgee jacket, this was to absorb the sweat that poured from their glands. The radiators seemed to be full of pyjamas warming on them. We had the ceaseless taking of four hourly temperatures, pulse and respiration. Oxygen was given to those who could not breathe without it. I often wonder whether it was any use but it gave the relations a feeling of comfort to think that SOMETHING was being done. The patient who was getting to the CRISIS, i.e. when the temperature miraculously fell and the patient slept to awake with the fever gone from his poor body, often became violent in delirium and had to be watched very carefully, as at night they were often to be met, running down the darkened ward, in a little short shirt. I feel the hospital authorities might had extended the length of material for these garments. This, if you happened to be alone on a ward was not only embarrassing but frightening, not only to the poor little Pro., or Pros. concerned, but to the other patients. As we had only one male nurse, and he belonged to the V.D. ward, on day duty, we had to send for the night porter to rescue us from this predicament.

Like the treatment for anaemia, this also was on its way out, in only about three years and streptococcal pneumonia was to be cured more easily than the common cold, which in this year of our Lord 1960, is still incurable.

Those patients suffering from gastric and duodenal ulcers were medically treated in much the same way as used today.

Sister West was one of the few sisters who taught us when making beds to start at the top of the bed and ensure that the patient had his bedclothes right up to his neck and was well covered.

It is curious the things which a patient may believe and relay to his cronies. One man as I was washing him one day told me, when I asked him his age: "I'm seventy nurse, and six years ago the doctors operated on me for my appendix, I was given up for dead, they took every organ of my body out and laid it on the theatre table and then put them back again, but I am still alive as you see." I felt speechless after this recital. I did not seek to enlighten him as to the number of organs there are, it would have spoilt the good story of his life!

We, as is usual in all hospitals, had our fair share of suicides. If it was a man who had committed this crime against himself and his people, he was watched at the bedside, if he was fortunate enough to be still alive. The person who was given the unenviable task was one of the local police. From his point of view, this had its advantages as it was infinitely better than walking the beat.

Policemen in those days and I guess they are all tarred with the same brush, were always glad to flirt with a pretty nurse. Many married them as at the time they had to have their prospective wives vetted by their superior. I think they were under the mistaken idea that a nurse carried a certain aura of respectability with her. As nurses are girls, oh well, girls will be girls.

The women had a watcher who arrived with a black dress and white apron. These she donned and then sat with the poor creature who had not completed their ambition to rid the world of their society.

Some of these people had gashed themselves and had been patched up in the theatre. On Bailey and Bannister we always admitted those with coal gas poisoning. I always felt sorry to think that they should have reached such a state that the only way out was to take their own life and even in this to fail

On this ward I came in contact with one of our honorary surgeons. You may wonder why on a medical ward this should be. He was a specialist in the removal of thyroid glands. This being the gland situated at the front of the neck which controls our life, is the core of our personality. If it works too fast, we become highly strung, apprehensive and the pulse rate goes up alarmingly and we become a nuisance to our selves and to our unfortunate relatives. If it remains untreated when diseased, the patient becomes exhausted as he uses all his energy for the lightest exertion and has nothing to replace it.

If the patient was fortunate enough to have a G.P. who recognised the symptoms, then he was lucky. He or she would reach 'Out Patients' and wait to be presented to our Great White Chief, Mr. Carver. By the time the patient had reached the cubicle where he was examined he would be in a flat spin.

When the surgeon had proceeded to look at his neck, which was sometimes enlarged, either one side or both, he would write a letter to the G.P. and give it as his well considered opinion that the patient should be admitted to his ward. He would tell the startled patient that he must prepare for a stay of a few weeks and some treatment, ready for an operation later. After a suitable interval, the man or woman would arrive on Bailey or Bannister.

Mr. Carver had his own particular routine for the patient who came in for this condition. Woe betide Dr. Pearson, or any of us who did not carry out his orders.

The patient would be surprised to find that he had to stay in bed and from then on would not be allowed even to wash himself. He had to be fed by the nurses and worse still he was not allowed to go to the toilet. All this was to ensure that the heart was in a resting state.

His weight was checked every week as was his basic metabolism, i.e. the output of energy at its lowest rest. He was given a very small rectal washout every morning. This the patient took to be part of the treatment, when in reality it was to ensure that the patient did not know when he was to be operated on.

Three weeks after admission the patient was given a rectal anaesthetic called Avertin. The strength of this relied on the weight of the patient. By the time the nurse had slowly given this the person would be asleep and was taken down to the anteroom of the theatre, on his own bed. He would be given a light anaesthetic and the operation performed and then he would be returned to the side ward and nursed as an ordinary surgical case.

This odd treatment was to prevent the patient being "worked up" about his operation.

The great man prided himself that he left no scar and if it was a woman, she would be able to wear an evening gown without a sign of the operation. This was indeed so, as the incision was closed with clips and removed on the third day, or sometimes even the second. At times a running stitch was used with equal success. It must have paid him to do this operation, as in this part of the country, many people suffered from this complaint owing to the lime in the water.

Mr. Carver was the type of man that a certain type of woman adored. He had a great many private patients and his manner to them was a mixture of admiration and patronage at the same time. The latter they did not seem to notice. He was tall and not so long ago had been blonde, was inclined to corpulency through over indulgence in the flesh pots of Egypt. As he was driven everywhere in his opulent looking car, this did not help.

He was reputed to hate any woman who was not good looking. As he made his living from them he had to hide his feelings, but when it came to the nursing staff it was a different proposition.

The theatre sister was just the type to suit his requirements. Very capable, blonde, with a smashing pair of blue eyes, black curling lashes, which she fluttered at him over the mask she wore when assisting him. Her brows too were of a delicate shape and a suitable darkness to enhance her rather rare colouring.

Legend has it that a new nurse from another hospital, like me in her second year, was sent to accompany a patient to the theatre before she could have time to don mask and gown he had stalked through in his pompous manner, taken one look at her, hurried through the doors and without troubling to lower his voice had, in a tone of deep disgust, said "Who is that, take her away and send another nurse, one who is good looking."

I cannot vouch for the truth of this but I think it is very possible. There came the day when I was sent to the theatre with a patient who was to have his leg amputated. I had to stay there as it was the rule that the nurse from the ward had to help the anaesthetist. If all went well the nurse could stand and watch the operation and combine it with a silent flirtation with the house physician concerned.

However, on this occasion the theatre porter, who was responsible for any heavy lifting, was for some unaccountable reason, absent. The great man proceeded to make the incision and turn back the flap of skin, which in the end covered the stump. He then went on with the tying of the blood vessels as he severed them. Then, as he was about to saw through the bone, he called loudly for the porter to hold the limb till he had completely taken it off. All eyes searched for the offending porter. As there was no one else in an unscrubbed up condition, his eyes fell on me. His rather prominent pale blue eyes were bulging with wrath but having spied my 5 feet nothing, and my 7st 3lbs I knew that I was doomed. "Come and hold this D*?*! leg," so I did. As the limb was amputated well above the knee, this was an ordeal for me. My arms were nearly breaking, when to my relief the porter returned, so I gratefully relinquished it to the proper custodian. I thankfully returned to my place with the anaesthetist.

The patient returned to the ward and was soon able to be sent home, where he had to set to work and renew his life in a different way. At least the pain which he had suffered would be gone.

Another time I accompanied a woman who was having the operation for the removal of her gall bladder. Like a lot of women who suffer from the effects of gall stones, she was grossly over weight. Usually after the operation was over and the dressing strapped in place, it was the duty of the anaesthetist to help the ward Pro. to bandage the patient, which is known to the Medical and Nursing Fraternity, as a many tailed bandage.

This particular time, the skin sutures were being inserted when suddenly I became aware that the anaesthetist was in a bit of a flap and a fluster. The patient had for no apparent reason decided to be in a state of collapse. Under his supervision, I gave a heart stimulant called Coramine and she gradually recovered but he could not leave the patient's head. So there was I, without help. Theatre sister and the big white chief were peeling off their gloves and his assistants had disappeared. So there I was, struggling to reach from side to side of the patient's mountainous abdomen. I had to stand on a stool. At last it was nearly adjusted and I became aware that Mr. Carver was beaming down at me. After I had pulled the last strap in place and at the same time made a fairly creditable imitation of the figure of eight, so dearly loved by tutors and first aid instructors, he said, "good little girl," and, if you can believe it, patted me on the head as though I was a pet dog.

The theatre staff nurse was a girl of twenty two, she had not long passed her State Final and was having a year in that theatre. Her face was round, and at first glance appeared to be childlike. Her hair, which was straight and cut with a fringe, enhanced this impression. It was only when one looked into her greeny grey eyes with their overcast long lashes that the impression was soon dispelled. They were hard, greedy and shrewd. Her figure was good and she knew how to use it to good advantage. She was a good theatre nurse but I fear that she had no liking for the chores that accompany the process of placing "the cooling hand to the fevered brow." She wasted not her time with portly, middle aged Honoraries, she was a good time girl, no more, no less!

Then there arrived at the hospital a house surgeon who was any young girl's dream. He was reputed to have a title, if this was true I never knew the name of it. Gerald, his name was. Gerald Thorne and he was six feet in height, athletic looking, dark haired and his eyes were blue as the Mediterranean is reputed to be. His lashes were long and straight and were the envy of all the nursing staff.

As soon as Clarrisa set eyes on him, apparently, his fate was sealed. Therefore I think she met her match, for he was equally unscrupulous as she was. They went about a lot together and as usual, rumour was rife. They openly made love with their eyes, their glances met and melted over the masks and from beneath pudding basin caps.

Came the day when they had been away for a weekend together and as Gerald's father supplied him with plenty of cash, they enjoyed themselves. At least they gave the others that impression.

At the end of his six months, he disappeared, leaving Clarrisa alone, minus fathers dublooms, minus the most handsome, conceited Houseman it had been my lot to meet there.

Clarrisa did not repine for long, she finished her year as staff nurse and took her charms off to a local nursing home, which was owned by one of the younger honoraries, not portly, but plenty of this world's goods. She proceeded to wreck his marriage for him, and when his wife obtained a divorce, she married him. There is a fool born every minute of the day.

Mr. Carver had the name among the medical staff for tackling operations which no other man would attempt. He was well named "Carver", but for all his pomposity, there are many people alive today who have such as he to thank for their existence. Not many would take the risk. The larger the growth, the greater the challenge to his operating skill.

As there was very little treatment for shock in these early days of the thirties, the patient often died from this.

Whilst on this medical ward we admitted a man who had been diagnosed as having an aneurism of the oesophagus. This condition caused it to expand like a balloon and in turn made a false stomach, without the churning movements and digestive juices. This forced the patient to regurgitate most of his food.

The man whose name was Charley Wood was fifty years old, thin and emaciated looking. When he had been seen in O.P.D. by the great man, he had it explained to him that he could have the choice of two treatments. He could have a minor operation and have a permanent tube inserted in his stomach, through which he could feed nourishing fluids. This being a very doubtful way of spending the rest of his life. The alternative was to come into our ward and have extensive preparation and then to have an operation which was virtually an experiment at the time. A totally new technique in surgery, i.e. a small number of ribs would be removed and the oesophagus approached through the chest wall.

Mr. Carver had never tried this before as he had never found a suitable patient to take the accompanying risk.

Charley, when he was told this, thought of the matter for a while. Having considered the pros and cons, he finally came to the conclusion that the second arrangement gave him a chance of life and as he had no fear of the hereafter, he decided to take the risk. He was a bachelor with no relatives to worry about or to worry over him.

He was ordered stomach washouts, with soda bicarbonate. As I was well advanced in my second year I was allotted this task when on duty. This was an unpleasant experience for the patient, but he never complained.

As he was not bedriddened, he used to help other men in many ways. He fetched and carried bottles and bed pans for them, he took washing bowls round, emptied sputum mugs and fetched drinks. In all this he was quiet and unobtrusive. His tall, thin figure in its old and shabby dressing gown was a welcome sight to nurses and patients alike.

After Mr. Carver thought he was surgically clean, inside and out, he named the day for the operation. In books, newspapers and on television today they are always laying emphasis on DRAMA. This applies to anything connected with hospitals and staff. In my own experience, a nurse or a doctor is nearly always too busy with the immediate work in hand to appreciate that there is such a thing. In this case, it was quite different.

Charley was given his premedication at about half past one.

This consisted of injections of Omnopon as a sedative, and atropine to dry up the secretions of the mouth and help prevent asphyxiation. At two o'clock punctually he was wheeled to the theatre in his own bed. Sister left the ward to the care of staff nurse and went with him to theatre. I never knew a sister do this before, it was unheard of there.

After she had gone, the men became very quiet and talked in whispers and even the nurses went about their duties in a very sub-dued manner. We all had a feeling of emptiness and a sense of loss. Three o'clock came and went, four and then five passed. By this time the tension was so great that you could have heard a pin drop, and it stayed that way until five thirty, when we heard the soft drag of the chain, which acts as a conductor of electricity, hanging from the trolley. Silently, the porter, houseman and sister wheeled him into the side ward, which had been prepared for him. This all with the stillness that boded ill. Away went the porter and the houseman and the trolley. Sister called to me. I went. There was the result of mans pitiful efforts to alter fate. Charlie had died! The operation was successful, but the patient died.

I can only hope that the mutual courage of surgeon and patient has pioneered the way to more success with some other unfortunate in a like condition.

CHAPTER 14
"You Will Go To The Matron!"

Soon after this, I read one morning, with a certain amount of jubilation, that I was to be transferred to O.P.D. This department was well away from the hospital main block and had a tremendous hall in which the presiding genius was the porter. On no account could this department have been run without him.

In appearance he resembled Tony Weller, Sam Weller's father "the old 'n". He was in his late fifties, his face was very red, almost mottled at times, his eyes grey and bulging, his head covered with a crop of grizzled hair and last but not least a stentorian voice, which he used to no mean advantage. He made no difference to whom he directed his voice, whether it were houseman, patients or nurses. His green uniform with its row of war medals was so tight that he appeared to be poured into it. After all these years I still have a photo of him taken at the Christmas party given for the children. His brass buttons look as though they will fly off with a bang. After he had called out a few names he used to wheeze as he shouted, and cough and wheeze at the same time and bellow like a town crier.

My jubilation was turned to despair as I recognised my old enemy Ginger. She was ensconced there as staff nurse. I had not bargained for that situation.

The sister of the department was a small Welsh woman, with snapping slate coloured eyes. I found her to have a very erratic temper and little patience with slow pupils or those like me who merely made an occasional mistake. When she was annoyed she nattered on and on, and on, or should I say RAVED.

Simultaneously with my arrival in the O.P.D. there came a new houseman named Terrence Gordon, commonly known as Terry Garden. It was a few days before I became aware of him. One afternoon I was struggling to put on a rubber apron, preparing to assist in the small room that was used for plastering ambulant patients. I was tired and teatime seemed to be a long time away. Suddenly I felt the two errant tapes taken from my fingers and in a jiffy they were tied.

Very taken aback, I turned round and there was Dr. Gordon smiling at me. Together we went to the plaster room and he quickly applied a Selby's plaster. This was a very light walking plaster, applied to the leg when a fibula was broken. I have never seen this particular one applied since but it was very effective as it was made of strips of plaster put on in the same way as for the beginning of an elastaplast bandage for varicose veins. Then, instead of putting the bandage all round the leg it was bound at the top of the leg and above and below the fracture and once round the foot. It was not as weighty as the usual one.

While he was performing this task I noted that he was of medium height and appeared to be slim. He had very dark hair, twinkling dark brown intelligent eyes. He sported a toothbrush moustache.

He was in his element, I discovered later, when he was caring for children. I often wondered whether his maternal instinct made him look after me, as he did. As I was small and appeared much younger than my years.

For most of my stay on O.P.D. he was generally on hand to help me in many things. I found that he was a good doctor, with an almost uncanny power of observation. He was a great help to the patients, especially when shyness or diffidence prevented them telling the symptoms of their illness. He had a kind and gentle touch and was much in demand by the children and their harassed mothers.

He looked after me in the same way as a mother does a delicate child, and later, when I was transferred to other wards, he again appeared as unobtrusively as ever.

To return to the departmental sister. She was commonly known as Minny the Moocher. I don't know the origin of this but this name stuck like glue. It appeared to me that she was everywhere at once. As our waiting hall was so large and the consulting rooms all round, we sometimes thought to escape her but no! It was impossible. She was there when you least expected her to be. I really believe that she hated to go off duty for fear she would be missing something.

In age, she was about thirty five, which probably made her a little more anxious to cultivate the company of the medical staff. Unfortunately, they were not so eager I'm afraid, they only tolerated her. This was possible because she was a competent sister, even so, we had no option.

There was I, between two fires. Ginger on one side and Minny on the other. They both settled for me, as being their scapegoat.

If it had not been for Terry, those first few weeks would have been unbearable. It is hard enough to get used to an outpatients department, especially a busy one as ours was. They never seemed to leave the Pros. to themselves for a moment without Why? Where? and What? This went on till one day an incident occurred which, as far as I was concerned, put paid to a lot of nattering from Minny.

One Monday morning the waiting hall was packed with people and old Morgan, the porter, was directing traffic with his foghorn voice. All the patients sat there with what I should call their Monday morning faces. There were the old stagers, sitting waiting for their septic fingers to be dressed. There were new ones from the local engineering firm, with foriegn bodies in the shape of steel filings in their eyes. There were those, who had already before the week started, managed to cut off some part of their anatomy.

On this particular morning, Terry was not on duty, it being his long weekend off. Had he had been, this incident would not have occurred.

Minny was never very sweet tempered in the morning but on this one, she arrived in an extra sour frame of mind. We concluded that her repeated efforts to enslave our New Zealand houseman were not yielding the results which she had hoped for. It was unfortunate for her, and for us, that night sister was a firm favourite. Mr. Stuart did not seem to be aware of Minny's existence.

It came to ten thirty and I was congratulating myself that I had escaped her sharp tongue, and that all was well. Suddenly my complacency was abruptly shattered.

I had been peacefully dressing a man's hand. She put her head round the side of the cubicle, took one look at my effort, and started to yap, yap, yap, wow, wow, wow! Why had I put that dressing on. Why? Why? Why? Now this dressing had been ordered by Terry on Saturday and this was to be applied till Tuesday when he would see the wound. I could not explain and she would not listen. As Terry was not there to defend me, I had the full benefit of her bad temper. All this with the patient listening, their ears flapping, not to miss a word. Finally! "You will go to the Matron to ask for a move." For once, Minny had overstepped the mark, for I silently reached for my cuffs, which even in a crisis like this, without which no self respecting nurse would be seen on the corridors. Having put on these articles of protection, I started to run out of the side entrance of O.P.D. and up the hill which led to the main block and the front porch. As I ran, so the tears ran also. Down my cheeks, unchecked. If you can imagine anything so undignified and unprofessional as a small young nurse RUNNING UP hill, her face swollen and her eyes bleary with crying, well I can't. As I ran, so appeared the R.M.O. he spread out his arms to demand what was the matter? but like Rachel of old, I would not be comforted.

By this time it was nearly eleven a.m. This may not mean much to the lay person, but to the staff in any hospital, it would have a sinister significance. The Matron's office is usually open between the hours of nine to nine thirty. This is the legitimate time for any interviews, pleasant or otherwise. No nurse would go after that, unless sent for.

I landed at the office door and tapped, a voice said: "come in," so I went.

Matron sat at her desk, her intelligent eyes looked a little startled to see such an apparition, at such an hour. An uninvited guest. "What ---- ----. Sit down, compose yourself and tell me the reason for this unappointed visit." By this time I had managed to control myself to speak. "Sister of O.P.D. sent me to ask for a move." The surprise on her faced now turned to wrath. "Tell ----", then she recalled herself and listened to my side of the story and then and only then, did I realise what a fool I was to have come, as sister had no authority to send me, for such a trivial thing. I began to feel a great deal better after that. She delivered a little homily to me and as I was going out of the door, the last thing I heard, was as music to my ears. Matron was calling O.P.D. on her own telephone.

I never knew what transpired but I worked with Minny for another two months, without any discord. Despite this blissful state, I felt that she never quite forgave me for taking her at her word.

However, Ginger made up for it, by keeping me up to scratch. She certainly did not approve of the attention given to me by Terry. She was not interested in him, as she had her eye on the latest addition to the medical staff. He was ginger like herself, tall, pale blue eyes. Came from Glasgow, as we were constantly reminded of each time he opened his mouth. His one claim to fame, I later discovered, was that he was one of the best anaethatists the hospital had ever employed. He was long, lean and lethargic, it must have been the ether. He went by the name of Bruce Blair. The ward nurses would heave a sigh of relief when he was on duty, as it meant that the patient coming back from the theatre, was in a light state of anaesthesia. They vomited less and came round more quietly and did not need to be watched such a long time. Those of us who had the task of trying to wash patients, give bedpans, take temperatures and even dressings, all in a given period, just adored him. He openly said that he tried to make the life of patient and Pro. that much easier. He succeeded.

He escaped the toils of Ginger with great difficulty but most of us felt that he was worthy of better. Her interest in him kept her mind from too much thought of me.

Every Friday afternoon we held a clinic particularly for those who had that depressing complaint, 'bad legs'. Most of the patients were elderly but of course there was a sprinkling of younger patients. Men and women whose life was spoiled by varicosed ulcers. These the result of varicosed veins. We were taught that those with radiating scars, were the after effects of the tertiary stage of syphilis, now, happily, not so prevalent.

All the doctors had one treatment, or so it seemed. This was to apply Elastoplast Bandages to the afflicted limb. It was the duty of the J.P. to take off the old one, clean the ulcer and cover it lightly for the doctor to see. He would glance at it and if still necessary, he ordered the renewal of the dressing. As by this time, I was often the one to apply this. It sounds a very easy task, but if the bandage is not applied with the same tension, it meant that the unfortunate patient suffered the torment of the damned for at least another fortnight. Sometimes, if it was comfortable, it was left undisturbed till the month had elapsed. I leave it to the reader's imagination, when I say, to put it mildly, the removal was not pleasant for patient or nurse. Despite the affluvid, this treatment was often effective. As there are people who are allergic to sticking plasters, in isolated cases this brought them out in a rash, which was most irritable and treatment had to be discontinued.

I always thought it as rather a pathetic sight to see the row of patients, patiently waiting with their legs in varying stages of undress. Most of us were glad to be off duty on 'leg day'. It seemed to me that I was always there for that afternoon.

Our gynaecologist, Jimmy James, was a Scot, tall, rugged features, greying hair, piercing grey eyes, which regarded his patients, virtuous and the not so virtuous, from under a pair of black over hanging brows.

Normally a patient man, I remember one morning when I was waiting in the inner sanctum of the clinic for him to send a patient in, to undress and prepare for examination. I waited for a long time, and as I had sent the last one back to the consulting room, I was puzzled. I was watching the clock in dismay, as I knew of the list of patients waiting outside, when suddenly the door opened and Jimmy stormed in. "Why has the last patient not come in to me." I looked at him in amazement. "There is no one in here," I said. "Yes there is," he shouted. "There is no one in the cubicle Sir, and if you don't believe me, look behind the curtains." He peeped in, it was simply empty. Out he went.

When the patients had gone, he came in and apologised to me for his state of amnesia.

I enjoyed his clinics, as he taught me as painstakingly as though he was teaching medical students. After I had prepared all his equipment for him, he would explain as he examined, thus I learned much that has been of use to me in the years since.

All kinds of women came to him. Women of all ages, from young girls of only twelve, to the old ones, worn out before their time with hard work, worry and yearly child bearing.

One morning a mother came to see him, bringing her young daughter, aged thirteen. She was the picture of childlike innocence. Her face round and her body in the state of plumpness, known as 'puppy fat'. The mother, who had done all the talking, was worried, as the daughter had been suffering severe monthly loss. Could the doctor help.

After he had examined the child, I cannot call her any other title, he barked at her: "Do you know that you have had a miscarriage". As she looked at him, just like an owl, he said, "Do you know that you were going to have a baby?" "No" she answered, opening her innocent blue eyes and that was all he could get from her. "Get dressed and come into the other room". She did

As I could see that the mother was a woman who prided herself on her 'respectability', I felt truly sorry for her, when brutally told the truth.

Once when he was lecturing us on the subject of V.D. He gazed at the class before him and as his beetling brows drew together he appeared to survey us one by one. It must have struck him from his vantage of years and experience, that we all had smug expressions to our faces. Sitting there in our immaculate white aprons, collars and cuffs and our faces to match. Added to the self-satisfaction, he must have read in our young and untried faces that we did not understand anything of life and the temptations that beset others. "When you attend to these unfortunates, do not draw in your skirts, as though you are creatures apart, for it is not given to you to know what may befall you."

Somehow, I have never forgotten this advice, and often wonder as to the fate of some of the girls who sat there and listened to what could not befall them.

From the attic of my memory, there were many pictures unfolding before my eyes. One of them is the morning that a commercial traveller came to the O.P.D. He was seeking the R.M.O. Eventually, when the doctor was found, he took the salesman into one of the offices, and it appeared to me that he was there a long time.

Much later we came to know the reason, and did not realise that, in the case of that unassuming gentleman, were samples of fluid, which proved to be one of the greatest boons to the Medical and Nursing Profession. It was the introduction by the manufacturing chemists, by the name of Rickets, well known for their 'washing blue', of the antiseptic known as DETTOL. This was made from their bi-products.

To us, who had known nothing but Lysol and carbolic, this was magic. No more raw hands. We were told that it could be put on to the skin in its neat state, this might have been a god-send at times. I think it was of especial value in midwifery.

The medical staff went mad over it. They used it for everything. Septic fingers, which previously had to be soaked in Epsom Salts were now immersed in a weak solution of Dettol. All round the dressing rooms were patients with arms and feet, legs and fingers, all soaking in the cure of all evils. The place smelled like a ladies hairdressers.

Naomi, who was on the gynaecological ward, told me that it was used there with equal enthusiasm.

Until the introduction of M-&-P a few years later, this became the best local destroyer of bacteria.

Also, while I was there in the O.P.D., I saw the beginning of the use of a new type of anaesthetic. This was known as Evepan and was used in the extraction of teeth, and "Painless Paul" went crazy on it. It was the fore-runner of Pentothal, which is in use to the present day.

The patient lay on the table, with his arm rotated outward. He was told to clench his fist a few times, then a small tourniquet was applied, this dilated the vein, and then the houseman inserted an intravenous needle into the chosen site. The patient was told to count and before he had reached five or six, he was asleep. The teeth were extracted, and the patient returned to the recovery room and 'came round' without any vomiting or unpleasantness, and saved much time for the Nurses.

As Christmas approached, the attendance at O.P.D. became very regular.

All the children knew that if they attended during the year, they would be invited to the party. This was the highlight of the year to many of them. In the year I was there, we decorated the vast hall, trying to brighten up all the dark and dingy corners. This we did in the conventional manner, dear to the heart of a child, after all they had never seen it before. Streamers, balloons and tinsel, coloured festoons from the lamp shades. A huge Xmas tree filled one of the corners and when this was lit it looked, as one of the little patients said, "a fair treat".

Terry Gordon and the retiring, shy houseman from the children's ward, did a great deal of the entertaining. Between them, they had created a creature, which was their conception of the Lochness monster, at the time very much in vogue. Then they used to draw the very tubby Santa Claus. This apparition had a great resemblance to Dr. Witherspoon but the children were not too critical, all they wanted was their present from the tree.

Santa was sweating away in his fusty robe and from under his equally fusty beard, issued stale jokes. To the children they were rare and new, and they shouted with glee as their presents were handed to the fat porter, and in turn given to the right recipient.

After this, the nurses dressed in the costume of sailor lads, danced and sang, and gave a very creditable concert, and, with the help of the housemen, this went down well.

After this, all the children were given some of the left overs, their parents came to fetch the little ones and the party was over.

CHAPTER 15

"The Flowers On The Lockers"

After my adventures in the O.P.D., I was sent to the women's ward. This was a surgical ward and took in accident cases which needed to be admitted.

Sister Padgett was a very capable nurse, but for my part, I never felt too sure of her temper. She had the snappy black eyes that I always associate with a nasty one. She was tall, thin and angular and when she was in one of her hustling moods, she appeared to be all cap, skirt and roller skates. She must have been born with a four foot rule in her hand, for her one obsession was tidyness. It appeared that she cared nothing about her patients, they were only there, only to please her symmetrical eye.

Naomi, who was and still is, more tolerant than I, said I was prejudiced, as she had worked with her and found her to be a good teacher and a very kind woman. However, it was I who saw her in another light. I felt that I should go mad if I had to work with her too long, as we had to tidy beds till I did it in my dreams. Tidy beds... tidy beds... tidy beds. After breakfast, after lunch, after and before dinner, after tea we made them. After supper and before we went to our own supper and so off duty. The only reason we did not have to do them before breakfast was that she was not there AND we had only just finished making them.

She would stand at the end of the ward and gaze down the length of it and woe betide any nurse who did not see eye to eye with her and had not persuaded all the sheets to remain exactly ten inches at the top of the bedclothes. Their fate was worse than death.

What the patients said to having half their chests exposed to the atmosphere of the east coast, I never really knew. They had too much respect for our innocence, I expect.

Her other obsession was lockers. These must be empty on top. Only a jug of water and tumbler allowed. All the patient's flowers had to be on the window sills or on the stack in the middle of the ward. This was sensible but the patients did not think so.

It was said that if a nurse offended her, she gave an adverse report to the Matron and also never forgot or forgave.

For a long time I remained in her good books but always with a feeling that I was living on top of an active volcano. However I was lulled into a false sense of security when I found, that my pedestal had feet of clay. I fell with a resounding bang.

First of all she crept around the screens when I was doing some minor treatment. Her eagle eye took in the fact that I was using this woundless treatment with a CLEAN towel, but NOT a STERILE one.

The final misdemeanour came when she appeared, I thought

she was safely off duty for the rest of the day. This was not really surprising as I think she hated going off duty, she was afraid of missing something. I think that her ward was her life.

This day, Mrs. Brown, in the second bed down the ward, had been very ill and on the danger list. She was now on the road to recovery and had asked me as a favour, that she might have the sweet scented flowers, bought by her husband, on her locker, till they were collected in the afternoon after tea. I felt the opportunity had knocked and I brought them to her. On her face was a look of content, as she gazed at this gift from her husband who adored her. I had the feeling of well being which comes to us all at times, in the most unexpected places and at the most unexpected times.

My feeling of elation and goodness did not last long. Suddenly, the doors opened and in walked Sister Padget. Her eyes snapped and the flowers were snatched from the locker, and I came in for the worst Yap! Yap! that I ever heard. Minny the Moocher was an amateur compared to her.

After this she only spoke to me if necessary and I was soon moved to the men's accident ward. On nights, after five days introduction to it, on day duty.

Have you ever tried to walk down a very long ward, bearing a tray of non-alcoholic drinks in your hands and this to the tune of 'Colonel Bogey'. Well, this it was my lot to have to do. Unfortunately, as the patients for whom they were intended, were at the wrong end, I had to walk the whole length, to the tune of the rousing march. I liked to deceive myself that I had the will power to WALK and NOT march.

As at the time, there were no very ill patients, only men suffering from mechanical breakdowns and they were full of repressions and therefore devilment. On thinking of the matter, through the mists of time, I have come to the conclusion that a tune, whistled with full force by thirty healthy men is not the best aid to help a nurse to appear dignified and professional and give a nonchalant air.

Having surmounted this difficulty, I stayed on day duty for five days, just in time to learn the patients' names and the general layout of the ward.

My first night on the ward had a slightly awkward beginning. It happened thus. Rosie Foulstone, my senior on this ward, and I, had jointly heard the report from the day sister. After she had retired, and between us we had done the evening treatment, and settled the patients for the night. I went into the sluice room to clear up, while Rosie took the four hourly temperatures and waited for the visit from the night sister.

There was a patient, who was convalescing. A handsome Romeo, tall and slim, with melting brown eyes. These he used to advantage all females from fifteen to fifty years of age. I think he thought that he was irresistible. As he was useful, to men and nurses alike, he was allowed to fetch and carry bottles and bedpans from the sluice room.

However, I was getting along very well and the chores were diminishing quickly, when in he walked, on some pretext or other. He picked a utensil from the rack and then proceeded to lean against the wall and make conversation. This consisted of trying to make a date with me, when he was discharged the next day. I had not even time to attempt to squash him when, night sister walked in. As the offender was looking at me in a most lover-like way, she could not be forgiven for thinking the worst.

Alas! I was in her bad books for the rest of that time on night duty. I was junior still, so this was not so surprising, as she had a reputation for 'getting it in' for an unfortunate Pro. of this rank. She would lead her a dance and then to the same nurses surprise, when again they met and she was a senior, night sister would greet her as an equal, with respect and completely changed manner.

Her favourite trick to catch the unwary Pro., was to inspect the sputum mugs in the early morning round, before the harrassed Nurse had had time to empty them. I hated this habit of hers and one morning, towards the end of my spell on night duty, I told her so, as I felt it was very unfair. Strangely enough, she did not make any comment, just told me to go back to work.

As I have mentioned before, Minny the Moocher, was running neck and neck in the marriage market. The prize being Mr. Stuart, the New Zealand houseman. In the end Sister Bebbington won, and finally became engaged to the doctor of her choice.

Apart from these minor incidents, I enjoyed all the time spent on this ward. It was a new building and much easier to run than the older wards. We took in all accidents from miles around. Most of the victims were airmen from the two nearby airdromes. They came not to grief whilst flying! They nearly all rode motorbikes, and at weekends they FLEW with their girlfriends round the countryside. The results, I leave to your imagination.

One officer, I remember, was admitted with a fractured tibia and concussion. His leg was put into plaster and a cradle over it to keep the weight of the bedclothes off his toes. For a long time, he suffered the delusion that he was a milkman. When the other men were snatching their last few minutes rest before being awakened to the tune of enamel bowls, etc. He would sit up and grasp the near end of the cradle and shout, in a stentorian voice, MILKO, MILKO, GLADYS? IVY? MOLLY? Having aroused every one, he would then become quiet. He gradually lost this delusion, becoming always surly and an ill tempered fellow.

Rose Foulstone was a blonde haired girl of twenty two. She wore with good effect the coveted navy and white spotted dress of the third year nurse. I enjoyed working with her, we had lots of fun.

She was even tempered and to look at here one would think that butter would not melt in her mouth.

Her eyes deep set and blue, and as a contrast to her natural blonde hair, her brows and lashes were black. She was easy on the eyes, or so the housemen thought. Here favourite was a pimply, nondescript youth from over the border. He answered to the name of McCowan. Beyond this I cannot remember.

Someone had once told her that she had bedroom eyes and she took it as a great compliment. She practised using them on anyone who stopped to appreciate them. At the time, it was the pimply one who was beguiled.

When we left the dining room, after our breakfast in the evening, it was my task to collect our meal cans. These were of enamel and were in tiers. Three of them. Each compartment contained different food, some cooked and others to cook.

When we were not hectically busy, we used to have our meal in the kitchen. It was forbidden to have them together but we did if possible. I would lay a nice cloth on the table and hide the deficiency of it. Having produced two fresh eggs from grateful patients and borrowed a vase of flowers, also belonging to a patient cut an orange in half to look like a grapefruit, add any other delicacies that could be scrounged. I would cook bacon and egg and we would dine in state.

We were allowed one hour off duty officially. This we took in turns, only if the ward was not too busy. We used to curl-up in the kitchen, wrap a blanket around us and sleep. Usually from two to three and three to four. We then had tea and toast and started treatment, etc. It was wonderful to sleep, but oh the awakening.

It was while I was on this ward, that a new experiment was carried out. Till then, patients in most wards were awakened at four in the morning. They were often washed at this unearthly hour, especially when we were busy and this was a chronic state. Those who were not on any treatment were awakened by the noise and lights of the other beds.

At this time, the committee and Matron and the other executives, had seen fit to alter this rule. From then on the decree that no patient was to be wakened till six a.m. and then, with a cup of tea and a biscuit, not only astounded us, but left us in that state which makes "necessesity the mother of invention." The only way we could circumvent this decree was to wake, one at a time, these unfortunates who were ordered dressings, enemas, etc. So at four thirty sharp, the screens were put around anyone who came into this category, the light over head was dimmed and we not only did their treatment, but we washed and made their beds. It made it a creepy business and deceived no-one, especially the patient. It was our only defence, for we were still expected to do the same amount of work, between six and seven, as we formerly did between four thirty and seven. I think we were one of the first hospitals to carry out this effort and I expect may others adopted this after.

Every night was not spent so peacefully. I recall one in particular. This evening, we came on duty to find that there had been admitted during the day five accidents. The worst one had happened to a young man of only twenty six. He was involved in the inevitable motor accident. Day sister reported that his leg had been hanging by a thread, so immediately he had been taken to the theatre and the limb had been severed completely. He had lost too much blood.

By the time we arrived on the scene, he was recovering from the effects of the anaesthetic. The shock had been terrific and we had not the means of combating this, as we have today.

It was the first time I had nursed anyone with an amputation, consequently, I was astounded to hear him complain that his 'toes hurt'. As he had no toes on that leg, I thought he must have been rambling, in delirium. This he was to do very soon. In the meanwhile, Rose explained to me, that the nerve that had run to his foot was still alive in his stump.

We could not explain to him that he was minus a limb, as he was not in a fit state to take it.

By the next night when we took over from the day staff, the poor fellow was in a very ill condition. He had already contracted the dreaded septicemia, which, we had no cure for. His temperature rose steadily, higher and higher. As the night went on he became almost unmanageable, in delirium. He shouted and tried to climb out of bed. Rosie and I could not cope with him on our own and do all the other work. But this is what was expected of us. So we rang for the night porter to help us. We then put some boards on the sides of the bed. These were well padded and for the night, effective. The houseman, pimply one, came and wrote him up for some morphia. This we gave and he quietened down as dawn approached.

Next night was even worse. We had several ill patients at the time, because we had had to take the overflow from Mr. Carver's ward. They were trying to paint the place.

By this time his delirium came from the muttering and restless state, to violent, spasmodic movements, over which we had no control. No drugs seemed to help him, Sister Bebbington sent the night runner to help in the late evening and in the early morning. In the meantime, we had to do the best we could. About two in the morning, he became so violent that he threw himself over the side of the boards. All this while we were trying to prevent it. We were not allowed to put any restraint, e.g. such as is used in mental hospitals. Not even a jacket with strong straps to tie to the side of the bed.

He flew over, just like a fish out of water and there we were,

Rosie and I, we tried in vain to lift him back, but all to no avail. He must have weighed about twelve stone.

I ran to the telephone and our long suffering porter arrived in haste. I had also reported it to the houseman and the night sister. Rosie in the meantime had tried to cover him with a blanket.

Having put him back into bed, he then went to sleep. The sleep of utter exhaustion. By the next night he had died.

Now, as we could not in any way have done anything else for this man, we felt badly about it. The next day, we were called to the Matron's office and had to go step-by-step over the whole incident and consequently there was NO NEGLIGENCE. We were exonerated from blame. I expect she had to face a committee, who would want to know the ins and outs of it.

The only blame was on the authorities who had not employed a male nurse to be a runner between the mens wards. I would like to know how anyone would have fared, had they been in the same predicament? Thirty four men to care for and one mad man, taking up all the time!

Hand in hand with tragedy, goes the comic relief. This one came in the form of Joshua Neil. Admitted with a mild concussion, he stayed with us for a few weeks. I was transferred to the isolation ward before he left.

He was tall and powerfully built, thirty eight years old, a mop of black, wiry hair. This was a mass of curls, which any girl would have been proud of. His cheeks were rosy and his eyes a vivid blue.

When he was first admitted, his bed was directly behind the desk in the middle of the ward. When our various tasks were done, and one of us having our rest hour, the remaining nurse would sit and study, read, or if the opportunity knocked, have a mild flirtation with the available houseman. Terry used his unobtrusive manner to arrive when Rosie was having her rest. He would always have a laudable reason for being on the ward. However, strange as it may seem, Sister Bebbington never found him. Maybe because Mr. Stuart was otherwise engaged.

One night, I was sitting there, studying for my hospital final, which was looming ahead. The ward was silent and all the corners in darkness. The overhead light shone down on my bent head as I tried to pursue the various subjects with which we were armed theoretically to face the world of nursing.

Suddenly, a voice called "Nurse"! I turned my head and realised it was Neil, trying to attract my attention, without waking other patients. I went over to him and what he said certainly was a great surprise. "Nurse Herbert, I have been wanting to ask you a question, will you marry me?" "I am a widower with two children, aged twelve and fourteen, I am a blacksmith, I own a smallholding, I have many beehives and to complete it all I have six hundred pounds in the bank". "Will you marry me?" "Don't say no."

To say I was taken aback was putting it mildly and at the time I was twenty two, I was in that age that thinks anyone over thirty is already in their dotage. I managed to make some excuse and put off answering the question.

I thought he would get over it, when his concussion was cured, but no. Every night, he persisted, even when he used to walk around the ward with his fractured humerus, in an aeroplane splint. When I eventually went on to the isolation ward, there he would stand in the court yard outside the accident ward. When at last he had attracted me, he would still ask me the same thing. I am afraid all the other men on the ward must have heard him.

As I had no ambition to become a ready made mother, I tried to be tactful. However, I was very flattered and thought he would be broken hearted at the loss of me.

Feeling that I must confide this tragedy to someone, I told Rosie about it. What was my surprise was when she started to laugh and could not stop. It appeared that he had been secretly wooing her at the same time. I think he wished to make sure that he had a nurse in the family.

I had been at the point beloved by Victorian authors, of coyly telling him that I would be a sister to him, when this blow to my pride came. To say that I was deflated, was putting it mildly.

We laughed often over this in the days to come.

There is somewhere a saying, which deals with the long arm of coincidence. I had a good example of this whilst on the accident ward.

One evening we came on duty to find that five men had been admitted during the day. I was walking down the ward, with a view to seeing the new arrivals. As I passed the first bed, I heard a voice say, "Hello Ruth". I turned in amazement as we were not allowed to address each other by our Christian names when on duty and the patient in the nearest bed had his head covered with the bedclothes. So I was about to move on when the new man popped his head up. To my astonishment, I recognised my cousin David. We were first cousins of the same age. He had lived in London, and I had spent the long summer holidays with my father's sister. Until I was fourteen, when my Father had removed all his family to the West of England, we had seen a great deal of each other. He had been as one of my brothers. One of our hobbies had been travelling around London on the top of the open buses. We saw the passing of these vehicles. To my mind there is no way of travel to beat it. However, I digress.

As I had seen very little of him during the last seven years, I was dumb-founded when he told me that he and a friend had been on a cycling tour, been run over by a car and had landed up in here.

The strangest fact was, that I happened to be on the ward to which he had been brought. In a hospital of three hundred and sixty patients, this was more than strange. However, I felt a warm glow of pleasure to see him there.

While we were taking in patients from Mr. Carver's ward, there was among them a person suffering from carcinoma of stomach. He had had a history of vomitting and losing weight. He had been taken to the theatre and had a laparotomy (opening of the abdomen) performed on him. Even Mr. Carver's assurance failed him and he had inserted a tube, which enabled him to have a funnel attached at meal times. Then he was taught how to run in nourishing fluids. As you can well imagine, this was no way to have to live. Despite all this, as a handicap, poor George Perkins, both before and after his operation went about the ward. He fetched and carried for those who were bed-ridden and never was there a word of complaint from him.

He was only confined to bed for a few days and during that time, we did not know that there was any difference between him and the other men. We found that he had carried with him a great secret all his life. He was a hermaphrodite. Part man and part woman. After this we took notice that his voice was very high and squeaky and we then understood his acute embarrassment at having to be nursed with all the intimate treatment, which the poor male, when incapacitated, had to suffer from the "young girls", as we were called by elderly men. This in tones of deep disgust.

George told us, that he had been a Regular in the Army and had served in the South African War and had been an "Old Contemptable". How he managed to keep his secret, I do not know, but history has it that many women have masqueraded as men and have been through and preserved the secret of their sex. I then had to presume that George, as he had been baptised, had done the same.

To me, this was one of the greatest tragedies that I had as yet, come into contact with.

When he had had his sutures removed he returned to his lonely existence, in digs. We knew that it was only a matter of time before he would have passed from the world and all its attendant worries.

CHAPTER 16
"Back On The Isolation Ward"

Just before I left this ward, Gwyneth Price was transferred to us. I had the satisfaction of seeing her, on her first morning and before we went off duty, carrying a tray down the centre of the ward and hearing Colonel Bogey whistling Da! da! da! da! da! Poor Gwyneth was doing her level best NOT to march, she was sweating in her supreme effort.

She was a dark haired, plump girl, with dark eyes and a happy-go-lucky disposition. She appeared to be in the perpetual state of breathlessness, which caused her to look as though she was shredding a cocoon, as her uniform never seemed to fit her and was in a continual busting of the seams.

As she marched, her good nature made her laugh and wheeze at the same time. She became a prime favourite with the men. She loved the men and the men loved her.

As I had been at St. Anthony's for a year, I was then classed as a second year nurse and so could don the coveted uniform, of white spots on a navy background. This was worn with a white belt. The first time I wore this, was a day of excitement. The Pro. concerned was pinched in all possible places and at all possible times. This by all and sundry. The housemen, in particular, made the most of their opportunity. Especially if she was a buxom blonde.

After this honour was conferred on us, we were known as the Junior Staff Nurses. I always remember one maid, who had previously worked in a mental hospital and had a habit of addressing us as "Staff". "Yes Staff, no Staff!" For some reason, this type of address irritated us. At this stage of our nursing education, we were expected to be a shining example to those who were under us. This was at first very edifying, but at the time became subtly depressing. Also, there was the Hospital Examination looming in front of us. Our examiner was well known. She had written a book from which we had to study. This, though full of instructions, which the perfect nurse, not yet found, would try to memorise, if not completely to practice.

At this time, there were a number of nurses off sick. There was an epidemic of flu. I had not succumbed, but Naomi was one of the unlucky ones. Our sick bay was full. In the next bed to Naomi was a girl by the name of Marjorie Kennedy. A pretty, slim, fresh complexioned girl. Her hair was dark and naturally curly. Normally lively and cheerful and full of fun. After she arose from her sick bed, she like the rest of the sick staff, were allowed the very minimum of time to recuperate. They were hustled back, as fast as their shaky legs could take us.

Naomi thought that Marjorie needed a little cheering up as

she seemed depressed. So I suggested to her that we went out for a day. We went to our usual restaurant and then on to see the film that was then showing. This one was highly appreciated by me, as it was full of rather sickly sentiment. After this royal entertainment, we returned to Lyons for tea and then back to the hospital. As I said "Good night, see you in the morning", she stood at the bottom of the little flight of stairs and just nodded and did I imagine it, or did I hear her say "perhaps?" I waved and went on my way, thinking of our conversation which had revolved around her boyfriend in London, the latest dance and how one of the oldest physicians, reputed to be well over seventy, had danced the Polka with his coat tails literally flying, as he danced with Sister West, from the medical ward. We agreed that it was funny, especially as we were used to seeing him with his favourite machine, an ancient Electrocardiogram, this he wheeled to the patient's bedside. When the patient became used to this fearsome object, it gave him a feeling of superiority and was a source of conversation with his relatives, when they came to visit him. I expect he knew more of this procedure than ever I did.

I went, after I had had a bath, to bed. When I came to breakfast next morning, I was aware that the atmosphere was charged with a certain tension. The room was full of silence, yes, it felt like that!

When at last I had penetrated the mystery, I was horrified to know that Marjorie had committed suicide, by hanging herself with a piece of extension cord taken from the accident ward.

At the inquest, it was said that she had no worries of any kind, was very popular with the nurses and altogether was a likeable character.

I still have a photo of a crowd of trainees and Marjorie is with them. When I look at it I feel that the only indication to the morbid streak in her, was her eyes, which were a little close together.

Most of the third year nurses who were due, like myself, to take the Hospital Final, had a particular dislike for this one. The reason being, that they had to converse with the author of this awe-inspiring and learned book, which they had to study in order to know some of the antiquated treatments, e.g. mustard poultice, linseed poultice. These had gone out many years before. I was lucky, I had not yet taken an exam with her, as I had had mine at the W.G. I never minded taking ANY test, as I always felt that it was a challenge to me and therefore treated it in the same way as an adventure.

However, as it was a few months away, I prepared to enjoy my holiday, which I took rather earlier than usual. I went for three weeks. When I returned after having a glorious time, it happened to be my birthday, also it was a warm, sultry day and altogether I felt somewhat depressed.

I had arrived very late in the afternoon and there did not appear to be a soul in the nurses home. All this combined to make me feel neglected, no-one loved me, no body cared. I felt this was a good excuse to have a good wail and this is what I was doing when the door opened and there stood Sister Charlesworth. In a most concerned manner, she asked me the reason for all this misery. I felt very foolish, but had to make the most of it. So, I told her of my sorrow at having to leave my home when I had wished to have my birthday there. It was the lamest excuse I had ever heard of, but it was the best I could do.

Almost, without a word, she went. In about ten minutes she was back, bearing in her hands, a tempting tray of tea, sandwiches, and a miracle in the form of an iced cake, the nearest approach to a birthday cake, that could possibly have been produced in such short notice. Soon, Naomi and some of the others came from the wards and they helped me to enjoy a feast.

If ever this sister reads this book, I hope she will know that I never forgot the kindness and UNDERSTANDING shown by her to me. In such small ways, it is possible to make another life more happy.

Having examined the list of transfers on the notice board, I was delighted to find that I was booked for the mens surgical. This was an old fashioned ward, built on the same lines as the womens ward, run by Sister Padget.

Oh! What a difference, in the atmosphere. Sister, was one of the most pleasant women to work under and she was popular with patients, nurses and doctors. A tall, angular figure, with a lovely complexion, grey hair and blue sparkling eyes. In age she must have been about forty. She had been baptised as Patricia Linda Ewert. The Right Honorable Patricia Linda Ewart, to give her her full title. The only one she cared about, was the plain nurse, or sister. It was rumoured that she had suffered a great loss at some period of her early life. She certainly had the true sympathy for all and sundry.

Like Sister West, she cared little for Red Tape. She desired that the men should be comfortable. Her nurses happy. My idol Mr. Barber, had several beds in this ward, the greater number belonged to him and Terry Gordon was the houseman.

I think it was one long mad rush from early morning, till we eventually went off duty, at night. There was no Ginger to hurry me and I enjoyed every minute of it. I learned more about the practical side of surgery than at any other time during my stay at St. Anthony's. I learned how to do dressings as painlessly and quickly as possible. Having had lectures from him and remembering his cry, "Handle the tissues as little as possible". Literally, we never touch a wound but that was not the only thing. I learned the method of exposing the tissues, only at the last minute, when all the apparatus was ready.

I learned so much that was of interest to me, that I could not possibly tell it. I learned the value of co-operation between the surgeon, sister, nurses and housemen. This ward and it's staff were the best example of it.

Everything was for the GOOD of the patient.

I have always loved the stir and bustle of the surgical ward, and with good team work, it is very rewarding.

We reserved the end of the ward for patients who were suffering from complaints of the bladder and kidneys, or collectively 'water works', a large percentage of whom were elderly men, who often had enlarged prostate glands. They arrived to us with distended bladders and were in great pain. The first thing, in this predicament, was to insert a self-retaining catheter and very gradually reduce the distension. This method was adopted to prevent shock, which would be dangerous, if the bladder was emptied quickly. The men were confused, owing to their complaint, and to the fact that they had been removed from their normal environment. This explained the reason that the night nurse might walk down the ward, probably congratulating herself that all was well, and promising herself a cup of tea, when her dreams would be rudely shattered, for there, sitting up in bed, in the half light, she would see old grandpa Digmore, waving a snake like object in his hand. This proved to be the catheter. When this appeared, the luckless houseman was supposed to come and insert it again.

These "Water Lilies", as they were disrespectfully called, deserved their nicknames, as far as they had an operation for the removal of their prostate gland, it became an exceedingly damp business, for the patient and made a great deal of work changing wet sheets for us. Not only did the patient have a catheter inserted, into his bladder, via his abdomen, but he was harnessed to a contrivance, which was known as Hamilton Irvings box. I will not attempt to describe this invention, but sufficient to say, it gave grandpa something else to wave, if he could.

The surgeon who performed this operation was know as Pa McAtheter. I never knew him by any other name. He was middle aged, tall and thin. Much like a drooping lily himself. He appeared to have all the cares in the world. I never saw him smile and his voice was flat and dull. For all these deficiencies, he was a patient man, and his "water lilies" did well under his treatment.

As we only had one male nurse in our hospital, we did treatment that now-a-days would only be done by a man.

This character was known as Carstairs. He was State Registered and had taken his training at an unknown hospital, unknown to us, he was the right hand of the V.D. clinic and ward. This block was known as Washington Ward. The indoor entrance to this was one of the main corridors, for staff only. Many a time have I seen Carstairs emerge from the doors, dressed in a stiffly starched coat, all shining and white.

In one hand he would be carrying the tackle for shaving the men in preparation for their operation. If his left arm appeared to be somewhat stiff, it would not be because he had rheumatism, but it was owing to his habit of carrying gum elastic catheters inserted up the sleeve of his coat. Should one of the men require catheterising, he would produce one like a rabbit from a hat and with no more of ado, proceed to do his worst. Strange as it may seem, his patients came to no harm. If one of us had escaped the diligence of the sister and had had the temerity to do the same, I am sure that every micro-organism possible would have invaded the unfortunate patient and our superiors would have had us hounded out of the place.

One morning when I awoke, I jumped out of bed and immediately came to the conclusion that this was not my room, but the Bay of Biscay and I was a passenger in some ill fated ship. The floor was heaving in a most peculiar manner, so I sat heavily down on the side of the bed and debated. I then came to be aware that it was the state of my legs, not the floor. The latter were made of jelly.

Eventually, I fought a battle with the buttons of my uniform. With difficulty, I mastered them and staggered to the dining room and thence the ward. I was not off duty till evening, but having survived most the day until the afternoon, staff nurse became aware that what she took to be stupidity, was caused by illness. She rang the R.M.O. and told him that she was sending me to casualty for him to 'ward me'.

I took myself to the appointed place, wrapped up in a cloak and sat shivering, with my throat burning and my head singing. I waited and waited, finally I must have dozed, for I awoke with a start to see our New Zealand houseman standing looking down at me. Seeing that I was huddled in my cloak and in a thoroughly miserable state, he put one finger under my chin, tilted my head back and commanded me to open my mouth and say Ah! in the traditional manner. He took my temperature and gaped at the thermometer with horror.

"How long have you been here?" I looked at the clock and I must have been there for an hour. He swore to himself, rang Sister Charlesworth and in a few minutes I found myself on the isolation ward tucked up snugly in bed.

I found that there had been some muddle and as it was weekend duty the R.M.O. was off. He was furious that I had been left so long alone and it was then only by accident that he had discovered me there.

Now, by an irony of fate, it was night sister's weekend off and

Minny the Moocher was deputising for her, as was the custom. She was by this time, fighting a losing battle for the affections of the colonial doctor but being of a persevering nature, she had not given up hope.

I remember little of what really happened, but only know that Mr. Stuart came during the night to see me, about three times. Don't harbour any false ideas about our houseman, he came to look at my chest and back and it took him all night to decide that I had NOT got scarlet fever, merely tonsilitis.

Every time he came, Minny came too. I really think she thought he had fallen for me, as her slate coloured eyes grew smaller and more black with fury.

However, she said nothing. Ever since my visit to the Matron she had been most careful in her manner to me.

I was off sick for a week in isolation, and from thence, I went to our convalescent home, about ten miles away.

When I returned, I was sent to the isolation block on night duty. This ward was usually given to the junior staff nurse, as it was a fairly responsible position. She worked alone, except for an hours help by the runner, which usually came in the morning.

The ward consisted of eight single cubicles, with a kitchen between. At each end of this line of cubicles, there was a room which took four patients. One ward for men and the other for women.

There was a passage on the inner side and a balcony on the outside. The nurse could see into the rooms through the glass windows of the passage or balcony.

It was a rather spooky ward at night and was not popular with the nervous or the superstitious. As I am not in either category, I did not mind. It is rather strange, but several unusual incidents occurred whilst I was there.

Whenever possible Terry Gordon kept me company. On those occasions he would wander round the kitchen and hunt around the pantry for tasty scraps, armed with these delicacies he would proceed to make a plate of sandwiches. If he had time he would help me devour them, if not he would make some coffee and depart to his own patients. I can only presume that he thought I needed care and attention and feeding.

Even though I was not in a senior position, the night sister treated me as an equal. I could do no wrong.

All patients who came into this block, had contracted some infection as a secondary condition to the one with which they were admitted.

They consisted of measles, with sinus trouble, women who had contracted the dreaded puerpural fever, which in those days could only be helped with good and skillful nursing and persistent treatment.

Their temperature fluctuated for days, often they were delirious. With all the care that we gave them, I am sorry to say that often they just faded out. I am glad to say, that now-a-days, if a woman is unfortunate enough to contract this, it can usually be controlled by antibiotics.

In the end wards were men or women with skin diseases. These meant long stay affairs and the poor patient was as heartily sick of himself, as we were of the constant changing of dressings. I think, even in the present day, that the patient with any one of the many skin disorders, is not to be envied. Many times it is tied up with allergy and psychological reasons.

Each patient was nursed under the Barrier System. At night there was only one nurse so you can well picture, that it was not easy. In every ward there was a gown, rubber gloves and masks. These were donned on entering the room and taken off each time.

One evening I had finished my routine work and was waiting for the night sister to do her round. She was fairly punctual as a rule, so I was wondering what was keeping her. At last I heard the sound of someone climbing the outside stairs. No! It could not be she. Never would she announce herself by singing "Auld Lang Syne", and songs with unmentionable words.

The kitchen door opened at last and in walked Terry Gordon and our latest houseman, a handsome heart-throb by the name of Dr. Basintude. Did I say walked? They could not have walked if they had tried. No, they staggered in, each supporting the other. "Beer, we want beer", they cried in unison. "Tell us where it is, I know there is some as I ordered some for old Johnathon, shouts Basintude. By this time, I was furious and all the patients were agog. What fun, it broke the monotony for them.

The two 'unable physicians', then tottered to the pantry and found a bottle of champagne, belonging to a sick nurse, who was given one of the rooms as a private ward. This was the last straw and I not only stamped my foot but I snatched the bottle from them and they turned sheepishly and supported each other down the stairs. Five minutes later Sister Bebington appeared. She soon disappeared, I don't think that she looked too sure of herself. Her self control was good.

Next night, I was even more surprised, for Terry and Basintude appeared, bowed to me in a theatrical manner, handed me a box of chocolates and simultaneously said in a duet "we have come to apologise to 'little nurse' for our lack of courtesy last night."

Having said their piece, they bowed once more and departed down the stairs in a dignified manner. I was left speechless.

I had found the reason for this jolification and alcoholic celebration. Sister West was leaving and as she was one of the most popular with the doctors, they felt that it called for more than the usual party.

After they had finished their liquor and had hunted for more, they were ALL DRUNK, yes, everyone except our tall, mystery Houseman, who was either tea-total or had a much stronger head than the younger ones.

It appeared that some of them had gone round the hospital emptying all the fire extinguishers and generally making themselves a nuisance. To crown it all, some bright spark had opened the window above the entrance porch. They had then thrown everything out of the window, all except the radiogram. This the mystery man had managed to save, for the future housemen.

I never knew the entire result of this picadillo, but I can guess. Soon after, two of those housemen were missing.

One of my most heart breaking experiences, occurred when I was on this ward. At the time of which I write, there were no private wards. They were in the process of being built and were completed before I left.

The nurse who I have already mentioned, was in this block, not because she had any infectious condition, but just to give her privacy, which we gave to any nurse or any one in the profession.

She had had an abdominal operation and when they had investigated, it was found that she had an inoperable cancer of the bowel. So an opening was made in the colon, to relieve the distension and free the faeces, so that she was not in so much pain. This was called a Colostomy.

It was one of my jobs to give her an injection of morphia to make her more comfortable and give her sleep as a result. I usually waited till I had settled the other patients and had had all the drugs checked by night sister.

When all the chores were finished, I gave her the injection. This had the reverse effect than usually achieved. She became pain free, and then she sat up in bed, had a cup of tea, which I, contrary to all the rules, seated on the end of the bed, shared with her.

She had been a practising midwife in the town and she talked to me of her life in the outside world. She listened with interest to the story of my love affairs and heard all the gossip of the narrow atmosphere in which I lived. She was a woman in her middle thirties and if she had an inkling that her days were numbered, she never allowed any self pity to enter into her manner or voice. She was always optimistic and considerate for others.

During the day the staff were all kind to her. Sister did everything to tempt her appetite. Dainty dishes were sent from the diet kitchen and Katherine, as she was named, would with great cunning tell the nurse that she would have her meal later on, when she felt like having it. The food was never allowed into the sick room, but went into the refridgerator straight away.

Her only pleasure was to have a belated cup of tea, with me, after which I would dine in solitary state, not on the food in our can, but on chicken with asparagus, tender pink ham with salads, fruit and cream. I always took pains to tell her how much I enjoyed this, as it gave her much pleasure.

She stayed with us, till she died, which she did soon after I left the ward. With all the years between, I still remember her and her courage was of a quality not to be forgotten.

One night as I sat studying at the kitchen table, I had a repetition of that hated condition which I had suffered from when on the children's ward at the W.G., night nurse paralysis.

I sat with a bright light over my head, my cloak huddled around my shoulders. It was about three thirty in the morning, when life seems to be at its lowest ebb. All was as silent as it could be, when suddenly, I heard a patient call from the four bedded womens ward. "Nurse! I want a bed pan." Then once again, more urgently, but I could not move. After what seemed hours and hours, I felt a light touch on my shoulder. "I have given her the bed pan nurse". This broke the spell, I looked round and there was a convalescent patient, smiling down at me. She had to come to the natural conclusion that the nurse was tired and had gone to sleep. I thanked her, but could not offer her any explanation, she would have been forgiven if she had not believed me.

When reading through this book, I reach the conclusion that far too many odd things happened to me, while on this block. However, as they are true I shall have to continue.

The next one, is only worth recording as we in this country do not often have earth tremors, or earthquakes.

Two o'clock. Night sister had departed five minutes ago. I had been out on to the balcony and had remarked to myself how silent it was, eerie in fact. The stars seemed to be hanging low in the sky, as though I had only to reach and pick one, in the same way one could pick a cherry from the tree.

The next minute there was a low rumbling noise, as of a lorry in the far distance revving up. I went inside and to my astonishment the cups on the dresser hooks were rattling and swinging back and forth. This phenomenon repeated itself once more and then all was quiet with a sinister quality about it.

In the morning I asked if anyone else had heard or felt this strange occurrence. None had! The only other person who did not think that I was going round the bend was night sister, who happened to be walking through the underground passages to another block. She felt the tremor and had thought she was imagining things.

Later on, I read in the paper that there had been a terrific earthquake thousands of miles away and we had felt the effect.

I was not the only one with odd things happening, for

Gwyneth had been sent to the Washington Ward on night duty. Now this was what was called a single ward. This meant that she was on her own in this old building, devoted to those who had contracted V.D. To Gwyneth, this was punishment, as she was fond of company and hated being in solitude. There were compensations, as Dr. Basintude found time to visit his patients more often than was strictly necessary. The patients on this particular night were all asleep and the houseman was away, so Gwyneth had the bright idea of standing by the radiator, to keep herself both warm and awake. Unfortunately, it was too warm and too comfortable and there, Sister Bebbington found her, standing up, fast asleep. Enough said!

After this we devised a fool proof system, or so we thought. After night sister had left the ward, I would phone her and visa versa. One night I was delayed a minute or two, I picked up the receiver and spoke the simple words, "The old girl is on her way". A voice replied, "The old girl speaking." The receiver slammed down. I was temporarily petrified. Strangely, she never referred to it. She must have been guilty herself once.

CHAPTER 17

"The Finals At Last"

My troubles and trials on this ward were by no means ended. Naomi said she thought that I had a jinks on my shoulder. Nothing ever seemed to happen to her. Her reports to the Matron went through without any outstanding remarks from the presiding sister. However, she was always willing to listen to my tales of woe, or otherwise. I strongly suspect that even if she did have worries of her own, she would not blazen them abroad.

My next adventure, if that it can be called, HAD to happen when night sister was off duty. Once more, Minny the Moocher was there.

I came on duty as usual, took the report from the day sister, who seemed to be in a hurry. Her fiance was waiting for her and they were late. Consequently, as she wrapped her cloak around her shoulders, she said "The patient will be back from theatre soon, toodle oo" and was gone.

I had just grasped the fact that a patient, who had sinusitis, with the complication of measles, after he had been operated on, he had a severe nose bleed. He was now in theatre, having the damage repaired.

I managed to do a round of the patients and enquired their wants, when I heard the whine of the lift and in he was brought. He was only very lightly under the effects of the anaesthetic. With the help of the porter, I propped him up and prepared to stay with him till he had recovered enough to be left. I hoped and prayed that he would oblige soon as I had a lot of routine work to be done. I had asked the porter to tell Minny that I needed help but as the runner was in another theatre, I had to wait till she emerged.

Our ear, nose and throat surgeon, Mr. McGreggor had issued instructions that the packing was on no account to be moved until he had inspected it next morning. The end was strapped to his cheek with a piece of strapping.

Just as he seemed to be returning to this world again, I heard the inevitable call for a bed pan. I ignored it as long as I decently could. Then I dashed to the sluice room, collected the utensil, pushed it under the poor patient, in a most 'un-nursely' manner and flew back to the cubicle, where disaster met me in the guise of the patient waving yards of blood-stained gauze in the air. He had pulled and pulled until it all had come out. I have never fainted in my life, but if I could, I would have done then. I was genuinely horror stricken and shocked.

I dashed to the telephone and called Minny, who in turn, called Mr. McGreggor's houseman. He was little, dark fellow from Ceylon, very nervous and he did not improve my feelings.

The surgeon had by now gone home and was probably

dining, hoping for peace. This evening he did not get it. He was told the disgraceful news and promptly prepared to return to the hospital. In the meanwhile, Minny had let me have it and when Mr. McGreggor arrived, he chased up the stairs and into the cubicle. His good looking face was flushed with anger. "Who is responsible for this negligence?" he cried. "I am Sir", very meekly. He looked at me "and who was with you?" he snapped. When I told him no-one, he was more mad than ever. Not with me but with the system that expected young nurses to have a dozen pairs of hands and eyes that can see through brick walls and feet that are fitted with wings, like Mercury.

The boy was taken to the theatre and the damage once more repaired and he was sent back with a Pro. to sit with him as long as necessary.

As it was nearly time for the hospital exam, I was moved to the children's ward on day duty. I have always loved to nurse sick children, so it was a pleasure.

All the children who had inhabited the balcony and verandah for so many weeks, those with T.B. had been transferred to a sanitorium in the country. It meant that we had more beds for those who were acutely ill. When they had recovered from their operation, sister had them out of their cots and beds in the fresh air.

One morning as Naomi and I were passing under the verandah, two boys were inspecting all and sundry. We were dressed in mufti and we heard a piping voice say, "There's a lady". The other in indignant scorn replied, "Garn, that ain't no lady, that's a nurse". We hurried away, splitting our sides with laughter.

Among our 'set', was a Pro. named Clara Compton. She was a calm cold looking girl of twenty two. She was of medium height, slim dark hair, pale skin and washed out prominent blue eyes. Nothing appeared to ruffle her. She was self-possessed and her manner had an air of disdain, faintly tinged with smugness.

For some unknown reason, Clara and I were often taken for sisters and even mistaken for each other. This caused an unspoken antagonism between us. I don't know why, I can only think that both of us were two distinctive personalities.

Unfortunately, we were in the same set and were forced to meet. I never knew if she disliked me as much as I her.

Came the morning of our exam. This was held in our large lecture room. The sliding doors were opened wide to make plenty of room. On one side were beds with convalescent patients who had volunteered to be victims of our mistakes and indescretions.

The other side was ornamented with tables and trolleys laid out with an alarming array of basins and kidney bowls, gallipots and instruments. There were treatment trays, for the laying for enemana, douches, bladder washouts, stomach washouts, taking temperatures, etc. There were boards for the spreading of, even then, outmoded plasterers.

As my surname had its beginning at the beginning of the alphabet, I made the natural mistake of thinking I should be one of the first on the list. I was eating my breakfast, with a certain feeling of satisfaction that I should have the ordeal over by ten thirty. Clara too, looked as though the same idea had occurred to her.

However, our self satisfaction received a rude shock. At lunch time we were devouring our treacle and cheese, when one of the Pro's came in with the news that the examiner had decided today, of all days, to start with those names which started at the end, instead of the beginning, of the alphabet.

This made me think that perhaps it was not my lucky day. All day I had a feeling of impending doom and the weather did not help. It was thundery and dark and those of us who had expected to be first, were in a state of jitters. At last it was four thirty and we were sent for and our misery was at the end. Usually I enjoy exams but this was not one of them.

At the door of the lecture room I met Clara and in we went. I saw sister tutor at the other end of the room and I interpreted her expression to mean that she also was heartily sick of that day. She gave us a sympathetic and encouraging look.

I then had a good look at the examiner, who had written a text book which was counsel of perfection. She was a very unassuming looking person with pretty naturally wavy silver hair. I could not even guess her age. Her figure was good. I did not care for the look of her eyes, they appeared too observant. We did not feel like being observed, we were too tired. I had put in a hard days work before I had started this practical exam.

Clara and I stood in the corner of the room, trying to look as though we were not there. All to no avail. She came to us and as we made beds in pairs, she told Clara to make up a bed for a patient with diptheria. I was to help her. I could see by her rather poker expression that she did not know the first thing about it. By the irony of fate there was little I did not know about diptheria, as I had contracted it twice and therefore felt an authority on it.

As we were not allowed to speak, this did not help. I tried to attract her attention to the fact that no patient with this disease was allowed any pillows. None at all.

When Clara had made the bed to her satisfaction, the examiner came and inspected it and proceeded to ask her many questions concerning the illness. I stood in silence, while Clara told her all she did not know of it.

Then it was my turn. Would I make a bed for a patient suffering from cervical caries. I looked at her, and I looked at the bed. I tried to bring from the corners of my brain any thought that would give me a clue. This concentration yielded nothing. I knew that caries had something to do with teeth. Beyond that my mind was a complete blank.

Foolishly I did not tell her that I knew of no such disease, so I made Clara help me with an ordinary bed, arguing with myself that at least I would show her that I could make a bed.

She came and looked down when we had finished but did not seem suitably impressed. "What would you do to stop the head wobbling?" she asked. "Put sand bags", I said. The light had at last dawned, but too late. With my sluggish intellect, I had at last realised that it was a disease of the cervical column. This is usually of T.B. origin and we had not had any dealings with such.

From this ordeal, I went from bad to worse. I was next ushered to the bedside of a woman volunteer and told to apply a mustard poultice. I had never applied one in my life and what's more never wanted to. I knew that there was something missing but could not think what it could be, so I mixed mustard with water, and spread it on some lint and plonked it on the patient's tummy. I cannot remember what she was supposed to be suffering from but I cannot think that it greatly improved by my attentions.

It was well for her that the examiner came quickly, "take it off nurse, what did you make it of?", and to the patient "it stings, does it not?"

After this I felt that nothing mattered, I was bound to be wrong. I managed to test some urine, even the difficult test for typhoid, correctly answered some more questions and thankfully departed.

Prior to the practical exam, which lasted an hour, I had written a paper, the main question on the Nursing of Typhoid. In this I had excelled. So when the results came I had passed. Fourth from the bottom. It was a comfort to know that others knew as little as I.

When sister tutor read her remarks to us, mainly on our deficiencies, she had written, "the bed for cervical caries was carelessly made. I then told her that I had not known what the disease was. She snorted sympathetically and held her peace.

It is worthy of note that in our set, there was a heavy, stolid girl, by the name of Nurse Lymphatic, that being her nick-name. She was our Gold Medalist that year and had high marks in this exam. I had never had any dealings with her and had no ambition to do so. Junior nurses had and when the results of our State Final came through, there was only one failure and that one was Nurse Lymphatic. Those juniors purred.

Naomi took her Finals a few months after I had left. She carried out what she had to do. A week after, she joined her fiance in the West of England and after the banns were read, they were married. As I have written, we were to meet many years later, after much water had run under the bridges. She has read all this story and says that she cannot think how it is that I remember these incidents after all these years.

After the exhausting time I had had, I was glad to go for a holiday. When I returned I was sent to my beloved accident ward, this was the last lap of this my first long adventure in nursing. The ultimate goal, which was State Registration. By this time I was only waiting to be gone from the hospital and to try out my newly acquired knowledge as staff nurse.

How I reached this Shangri La and what came of it, belongs in another book.

There had been appointed to the ward a new sister. Her name being Sister Goodwin. She was a delightful woman. She was tall and had a very stately walk. This gave her a deceptive air of moving slowly, when in reality, she did more work in less time, than others who appeared to do much. She entered the ward quietly and gave the impression of calm serenity. She was a good administrator and a grand teacher. She was not one of those women who were convinced that they are indespensible. She obtained the best results from her senior staff, simply by the method of trusting them, without any interference. This was till such a time came, when or if, one of them proved themselves unworthy of such trust.

I cannot remember any discord while I was there. It remains to me a very happy memory of my last few weeks in training.

The only fly in the ointment was Ginger. I had always been haunted by her. She was senior staff nurse but as sister kept me on duty with her, I saw very little of my antagonist. Also she could not say much as I was now, junior staff nurse.

One evening there arrived a double accident. They were two young men, one had been driving the unenviable motorbike and the other the pillion passenger. They were in a very shocked condition, each had a portion of a limb nearly torn off. They were taken to the theatre and as one had a foot and the other his leg, hanging by a thread, these had to be amputated and the blood vessels tied. This was rough surgery, till such time came when the stumps were in a state to be covered with a skin flap and allowed to heal.

They were both twenty two years old. One was a male nurse in a mental hospital and the other a magazine artist, who became very well known a few years later. His glamorous damsels with long silken legs and his HE men in Harris Tweeds, graced many a popular front page cover.

They had always been friends from childhood and still were despite their diverse occupations.

In the mornings, after the operation patients had been prepared, it was the task of the senior and the junior staff nurses to do all the dressings. If sister was on duty, Ginger did one side of the ward and I the other. Charlie and Fred were on my side of the ward and when we were making beds in the morning, in a stage whisper they would say, "are you doing our dressings? Are you on duty?" If I said "yes" all was well. If I answered in the negative, there were loud groans. Ginger was very heavy handed and I often thought that her pastry making, if any, could not have been a success.

These two lads were the most cheerful of patients and as their stumps were like pieces of raw beef and had to be dressed every day with flavine and parrafin, I could not see what they had to be so happy about.

However, thanks to the teaching of my idol Mr. Barber, I had mastered the technique of dressing most things almost painlessly. The first thing to do was to gain the confidence of the person concerned. I was very sorry that I had to leave before they had their final operation.

Whilst we made beds, they would sing and as the other men were mainly mechanical breakdowns, they joined in. Gwyneth Price was on nights and before she went off duty, she would also sing in her lovely clear Welsh voice. I know that it was not the 'done thing', but it was a tonic to those men and did a lot for their morale.

Gwyneth was happy at her work but was at this particular time, extra happy. She was engaged to Dr. Basintude. This had to be kept a dead secret, this was why we all knew about it, till she had passed her State Final. Such love affairs were frowned upon.

Jane Brodie was beginning to show forth her Florence Nightingale nature. She was competent and absolutely sure of her self and after many more letters were added to her name, she became Matron at one of the largest provincial hospitals in the country. All this some years later. Even now, I read of her. Perhaps she does not remember the Pro. who pulled her up and down in the lift.

As for me, I was the only one who was not engaged to marry anyone. I had kept poor Terry Gordon off the subject, up till now, as I felt that at any time he would be breaking his reserve. Although I had begun to take him for granted and had accepted all his rather maternal ministrations, without too much gratitude, I still did not feel like being tied down to any one man.

The day came when I realised that Terry was going to acquire more knowledge in what is now known as pediatrics. I was nearly due to take my State Final, in fact it was only a fortnight away, when I had to face this adventure.

Thus it was that I let Terry pass out of my life, thinking never to see him again. However this was not so. I met him again after many moons had passed.

At last the great day arrived. We were to take our State Final, the ultimate goal of those years hard work, physical and mental.

This exam was held alternatively, at a hospital forty miles away and at our own. I was glad when our turn came, that it was an 'away' one. It seemed more exciting and made a complete day out. There were eight of us and we shared a taxi, as we had no other means of arriving there in time. I remember little of the written one but enjoyed the practical and the oral exam.

I think that I succeeded in satisfying the Matrons in the practical that I was a fit person to be let loose and take charge of other unfortunate mortals, when they had no choice.

When it came to the oral, it was really good fun. As it came to my turn to answer the tinkling bell, I was ushered into a little room where sat a little red faced rotund man, with a shiny bald head and a pair of twinkly blue eyes. I think he must have been a physician in a fever hospital, for immediately he began to ask me the incubation periods of various diseases e.g. measles, scarlet fever, varicela and others. None of which I knew. As I never would admit defeat, I answered something.

He looked at me and said "I think you are guessing, aren't you nurse." I agreed with him, so he changed the subject. To my great delight he switched to the subject which at the time I was well primed in. The thyroid gland! Thanks to Mr. Carver I answered questions appertaining to this minute portion of our anatomy. I knew all the signs, symptoms, treatment of Graves Disease, Myxodema, Goitress, etc. I hoped that he approved and I had made a good impression after all.

At the second tinkle of the bell, I was ushered into another little cubicle. This time the examiner was a young looking man, with a thin, kind face. He looked at me sharply and said, "You have already been in here before". No Sir!" Not so politely. He still seemed to be very suspicious, when suddenly, light dawned on me. It was Clara Compton who had already been in. As we were alike and both wore the rather unusual uniform of our hospital, it was excusable. I then explained it to him and all was well.

He asked me what ward I was on and when I said accident he seemed pleased and proceeded to ask me all about concussion and compression, comminuted and complicated fractures. Showed me various bones to identify and I departed well satisfied with my efforts.

I have thought since that a lot of this intelligence was wasted, as the State, at that time, only required the nurses to obtain over thirty per cent pass marks. I do not know if this low standard is all that is still required.

Going back to St. Anthony's, we conned over our answers. I think they all worried too much, as I thought it was not a matter of life and death after all.

We regaled ourselves with an extra special tea, went to a

show and then to bed. Having endured this ordeal and returned from it, apparently unscathed, we set ourselves to forget it for six weeks.

As it was getting on towards Xmas, we began to prepare for the decorations. Although I knew that I should have left the hospital by then, I set to work and employed Charlie and Fred and an elderly man named Harry, who was an 'up' patient, recovering from an injury to his ankle. I taught them how to make lamp shades of all colours and to my own design. They all worked with a will, as it helped to break the monotony for them.

One day Charlie called me to him and showed me a cartoon which he had drawn. It was a very clever sketch, portraying our most junior Pro. She was doing her best to help and understand an old man in the bed opposite. He was trying to tell her that his foot which was in plaster, was in pain. Like me, she found the local dialect harder to grasp than a foreign language.

However, there was our J.P. complete with long apron, hanging below the hem of her dress and the safety pin slipping from under her white belt, horror of horrors. She looked young, harrassed and worried. To crown it all, he had reproduced the exasperation on the face of the old man and to add insult to injury, there was the hairs sticking out of his ears, just like a pair of tom cat's whiskers.

Later on he gave this cartoon to me and although it has long since been lost, I still remember it.

At last, one morning, Matron arrived at the ward door, waving an envelope in her hand. Hooray! a thin one. This was a good sign, as it proved that there were no re-entry forms enclosed. Quickly, I opened it and there they were, the few words which should have made me as excited as the others were. All I could think was "well, I don't feel any different from how I did a few minutes ago." This seemed to me to be an anti-climax.

We then retired to the nurses home, to don our new uniform and go to the Matron's office to be congratulated. As there was one failure, we tried not to rub it in by seeming too enthusiastic.

After this, it was time for me to leave the hospital. I had just a week and I was going home till I made up my mind where to go and what branch of nursing I would take up.

Several weeks before, I had travelled to London to see my first Matron, at the W.G. I had asked her if I could return to do a year as staff nurse. She told me, that only on one condition would she have me and that was that I take the course in midwifery. At that time it could be taken, if you were S.R.N., in six months.

I had already taken a four year training and I felt more tired and unsettled than I realised. I decided against this advice and by this course of action, altered the whole course of my life. The adventures and mistakes that resulted, I will write of one day.

Sister Goodwin seemed very sorry to have to part with me and presented me with a beautiful handkerchief case, filled with lovely handkerchiefs. She said it was for taking interest in the decorations which I should never see.

It was nearly time for Charlie and Fred to have their stumps repaired. They presented me with a fountain pen. This was a present from all the men and the collection had been sponsored by them.

Then came the morning on which I had my last look at this Hospital, which I had come to love. When I arrived at the station, there, waiting to wave me off, were Harry, who was going home and had delayed it to wave me off and John Priestley, an ambulance driver who had always thought more of me than ever I had of him. I looked at them and my eyes smarted with tears, to think of them both, the one older and the other as young as I was, remembering to make the effort to be at the station, just for me.

Also, there were two housemen going to London on leave. One was Dr. White, he was a thin, earnest, pimply youth from North London and lived near the W.G., with short sight and thick lenses to his spectacles. The other was Dr. Basintude.

The three of us boarded the train and I waved to Harry and John and then they slowly disappeared out of sight. As the train gathered speed, I sat down and gave myself up to thought, but I could not foresee what the future was to bring to me. After a while I began to feel a stirring of excitement, I was off on a new adventure. All my life, I have felt this way. Bad and good. It was New. Therefore something to be met, enjoyed, or battled with.